FOODS TO STAY VIBRANT, YOUNG & HEALTHY

The Complete Nutrition Guide for Midlife Women

Audrey Wright, M.S., R.D. • Sandra Nissenberg, M.S., R.D.
and Betsy Manis, R.D.

CHRONIMED
PUBLISHING

Library of Congress Cataloging-in-Publication Data

Wright, Audrey, M.S., R.D., L.D., C.D.E.
Foods to stay vibrant, young and healthy: the complete nutrition guide for midlife women/Audrey Wright, M.S., R.D., Sandra Nissenberg, M.S., R.D., and Betsy Manis, R.D., L.D., C.D.E.

P.   cm.
Includes index
ISBN 1-56561-057-1; $10.95

1. Nutrition

Edited by: Patricia Richter and Jeff Braun
Cover Design: Garborg Design Works
Text Design/Production: Janet Hogge
Art/Production Manager: Claire Lewis
Printed in the United States of America

Published by
Chronimed Publishing
P.O. Box 59032
Minneapolis, MN 55459-9686

About the Authors

Betsy Manis, RD, LD, CDE, is employed at Hillcrest Medical Center in Tulsa, Oklahoma, as a diabetes nutrition specialist.

Audrey Wright, MS, RD, is director of the Father Walter Memorial Center in Montgomery, Alabama. She has served on the Board of Directors of The American Dietetic Association and its Foundation.

Sandra Nissenberg, MS, RD, is a nutrition consultant in Buffalo Grove, Illinois. She is a former staff member of The American Dietetic Association and its Foundation.

Dedication

We dedicate this book to the memory of our dear friend, colleague, and fellow co-author, Edna Langholz, who inspired, encouraged, and challenged us to write and share our knowledge and wisdom in this book.

Table of Contents

Introduction

Vibrant, young, and healthy! Active and energetic! Vivacious and happy! Do these words describe you?

If your answer is a resounding, "Don't I wish!" then this book is for you. In these pages, you'll find practical tips for feeling your best—now and for years to come.

The secret to healthy, vibrant living really is no secret at all. It just depends on what you eat and how much physical activity you schedule into your life. The rest pretty much relies on the genes you inherited at birth.

As we get older, we need to become more aware of the nutritional and the special needs of our bodies. And, we need to be aware of hereditary factors that affected our parents' lives. If heart disease, diabetes, osteoporosis, or cancer seems to run in your family, you need to be especially vigilant with the care and feeding of your body.

For instance, studies show that groups of people eating foods high in antioxidants tend to have lower rates of cancer and heart disease. So it is a good idea to stock up on antioxidant-rich foods such as sweet potatoes, spinach, broccoli, cantaloupe, strawberries, and citrus fruits. Carrots are another example of a health-boosting food. Just two large carrots or six baby carrots a day can reduce total cholesterol levels by up to 20 percent. We'll share more about the specifics throughout this book.

Learning about nutrition helps us understand the purpose of food, what and why we need to eat, and how we can use basic foods to help overcome any health challenges and obstacles we may face as we age. But, we need to separate food facts and fads from fiction. There's more information about health and nutrition available to us today than ever before. It can be confusing, but this book is intended to help you sort it all out.

Your Changing Lifestyle

Chances are that near midlife you have or will change your lifestyle. Whether you work in a pressure cooker, travel constantly, face an empty nest or a revolving-door family, your lifestyle helps determine how you eat. If you are like us, you want a lifestyle that promotes good health and provides you with the vitality you need to enjoy each day.

Health means much more than just the absence of disease. And the territory between "just not feeling good" and "feeling great!" is vast. Choosing the foods that are rich in the nutrients your body needs and getting the exercise and rest that you deserve will help put you into the "feeling good" mode. Minimizing stress can push you straight into "feeling great!" Managing your lifestyle and your foodstyle can be made easy if you remember just three little words: variety, balance, and moderation. If there's a secret, that's it!

Your Healthy Foodstyle

Each body is different and our needs vary according to a host of factors. That's why you won't find any "blanket" advice here. But reading this book should help you to develop a "foodstyle" that is just right for you. As you begin the process, remember that small steps can take us on big journeys, and simple changes in our daily meals and snacks can lead to large health gains.

Healthy eating should be a pleasurable, satisfying experience. Diets promise deprivation, and that's not what we are talking about here! You don't have to give up your favorite foods. Instead, you can adapt your food choices to a new style by making simple changes.

The Choice is Yours

Since the turn of the century, medical science has made strides toward prolonging life. A woman today can plan to enjoy her seventh and eighth decades and beyond. Her grandmother, born at the turn of the century, however, usually only lived into her 60s, and if she lived longer, the quality of her later life was generally not very active. Research about women's health issues is still scant, however, and we simply don't yet know all we need to know.

Most of us are quick to admit, however, that we are not in perfect health. Every woman has her share of aches and pains by the time she hits her 50s. It seems to go with the territory. In this book you'll find some healthy alternatives to help you live with the challenges you meet along life's way.

Our bodies are designed to serve us well at every age, but only if we use our brains to make good choices. When changes become necessary, like reducing our intake of fat or salt and increasing our intake of fruits and vegetables, we want you to have good information to help make the choices that lead you toward feeling great. When a choice is made out of a fear of disease, it tends to be short-sighted.

Helping you make positive changes based on good information, that's our goal. Having a positive attitude about health is the important first step. Then set some goals in line with that positive approach. Know the facts. You have the power to make the changes that will lead you toward vibrant health and healthy living. The choice is yours!

Foods to Stay Vibrant, Young & Healthy

1
Nutrition & Good Health

Everyone is skeptical. Information about food changes so quickly, most of us figure what's bad for us today will be good for us tomorrow. So why bother to make changes?

While it's true that much of what we hear and see about healthy eating is sensationalized and exaggerated, it's also true we've come a long way. We have lots of good, solid information about what we can do to promote health and vitality—even as the aging process takes its toll.

We know that the human body needs more than 50 nutrients just to handle basic human activity—growing, regulating body processes, and providing energy for physical activity. Women, in particular, have unique nutritional needs because of the hormonal variations their bodies experience. Many of these nutrients are manufactured by our bodies themselves; others, however, must be obtained from the foods we eat.

Carbohydrates, protein, and fat are the nutrients that provide us with energy—and they are the only nutrients that contribute calories to our diet. Carbohydrates and protein supply only 4 calories per gram of food while fat contributes 9 calories per gram. Vitamins and minerals don't supply any calories, but they are the regulators of many body functions and are essential for maintaining and repairing body tissues.

Carbo-Powered Energy

Carbohydrates provide the body with most of its energy. All carbohydrates are eventually converted to glucose, or blood sugar, which is the primary fuel our bodies use for muscle and brain cell activity. Glucose is carried through the blood to the cells. If the body has more glucose than it can use for energy, the excess is converted to either glycogen (which is stored in the liver or muscles) or to body fat (which, every woman knows, is stored all over the body).

Table sugar, breads, starches, pasta, dried beans, milk, fruits, and vegetables are all carbohydrates. Carbohydrates come in two basic types. The first are known as simple carbohydrates or sugars. Sugars are also called fructose, glucose, dextrose, maltose, lactose, sucrose, syrup, honey, and molasses.

Fructose is found abundantly in fruits, honey, and syrups. Glucose is also often known as dextrose, or grape sugar. Sucrose is commonly known as table sugar, beet sugar, or cane sugar. It is found in many fruits and some vegetables and grains. Lactose, which is milk sugar, is the least sweet of all the sugars. Maltose is only found during the germination of plants and so is rarely encountered.

The beta carotene in carrots and other foods can reduce the risk of various types of cancer and also reduce blood cholesterol. Just 2 large carrots or 6 baby carrots a day can reduce cholesterol levels by up to 20%.

Sugar alcohols, sorbitol, xylitol, maltitol, and mannitol are made from dextrose or fruits. They are often found in sugar-free chewing gums and diet desserts. You should know, however, that they are not calorie-free. They contain the same amount of calories as sugar, but are metabolized more slowly. If excessive amounts of diet foods containing these sugars are used, they can cause diarrhea.

The other type of carbohydrates, complex carbohydrates or starches, are found in breads, pasta, rice, potatoes, and beans, among other foods. All starchy foods are from plants, and grains are our richest carbohydrate source. Rice, wheat, corn, millet, rye, barley, and oats are the foundation for most low-fat diets, and for good reason. Potatoes, yams, and cassava are also major sources of starch. Legumes include members of the bean and pea families like peanuts, kidney, pinto, and butter beans, blackeyed peas, chick-peas, and soybeans. Each of these has protein and fiber in addition to its carbohydrate value.

Complex carbohydrates should be our first choice when we determine our foodstyle. Their health benefits for women are many since these foods are:

- low in fat

- low in calories

- high in fiber

- high in vitamin content

- high in mineral content

All of these benefits help reduce the risks for obesity, cardiovascular disease, diabetes, and cancer, among others. So, you can see, carbohydrates can be a woman's best friend, at least when it comes to foodstyle.

Protein—The (In)Complete Story

The majority of our body tissues are made up of protein. As the basis of life, protein is essential for growth and for all body functions. It is continually being broken down in our bodies and so needs constant replenishing. Protein is comprised of amino acids, the body's building blocks. Some of these come directly from food sources, others are manufactured in the body from food components.

Protein that comes from an animal source is called a "complete protein." Generally this kind of protein contains all the amino acids we need to make and maintain body tissues. Protein found in vegetables, on the other hand, is usually low in one or more of the essential amino acids. Thus we refer to vegetable proteins as "incomplete proteins."

Vegetable protein is more usable when it is combined with another protein within the same day. The protein can be from either an animal or a vegetable source. Popular combinations include rice and beans or macaroni and cheese. Most Americans eat about twice as much protein daily as their bodies need, so protein-deficiency disorders in Americans are extremely rare.

Fat Facts

Yes, our bodies actually do need some fat. It is essential. Fat helps our bodies maintain healthy skin and hair; it transports fat-soluble vitamins through the blood, and it regulates cholesterol levels. It also stores the body's excess calories.

All fats have the same number of calories per gram, but they vary in composition. If you want to follow a heart-healthy diet, for example, you'll want to cut back on the amount of highly saturated fats you consume. These are lard, butter, fat in meats, coconut oil, palm kernel oil, fat in cheese, and solid shortenings. Diets containing monounsaturated fats such as olive, canola, and peanut oils, on the other hand, seem to promote heart health.

Fat has traditionally been seen as the "bad guy." This is understandable since it has been linked to obesity, heart disease, and cancer. But some fat is necessary for good health. It is the amount and the type of fat we eat that gets us into trouble.

The Big Picture

The following chart lists the major nutrients our bodies need. Specific requirements and food sources are covered throughout this book, particularly in the appendix (page 229).

Basic Nutrients Our Bodies Need

Water

Carbohydrate (glucose)

Protein (9 essential amino acids)—Valine, leucine, isoleucine, lysine, histidine, phenylalanine, tryptophan, methionine, threonine

Fat (3 essential fatty acids)—Linoleic acid, linolenic acid, and arachidonic acid (which the body can manufacture)

Water-soluble vitamins—Ascorbic acid (C), thiamin (B1), riboflavin (B2), niacin (B3), pantothenic acid (B5), folate, pyridoxine (B6), biotin, cobalamin (B12)

Fat-soluble vitamins—A, D, E, and K

Major minerals—Sodium, calcium, phosphorus, chloride, potassium, sulfur, magnesium

Trace minerals—Iron, zinc, iodine, copper, manganese, fluoride, chromium, selenium, molybdenum, nickel, silicon, tin, vanadium, cobalt, arsenic, boron

Lots of Liquids

Did you notice that number one on the chart is water? We sometimes forget water is a vital nutrient. Over half the human body is made up of water.

Water is the medium in which most of the body processes and chemical reactions are carried out. It plays a major role in the intestinal tract, keeping blood moving and eliminating wastes. It also combines with fiber to increase bulk in the colon to prevent constipation. Additionally, it dilutes impurities in the urine, reducing stress on the kidneys, and regulates body temperature, providing cooling perspiration.

Sometimes you can rely on your feeling of thirst to tell you that you need more water. But sometimes you can't. So, we often need to remind ourselves to drink water. We need 6 to 8 glasses daily, that's 48 to 64 ounces at a minimum.

Water is found in many of the foods we eat, such as soups and the variety of beverages other than water that are available to us. Caffeinated beverages, however, are not a good source of water since these act as diuretics and increase urine production, depleting us of the healthful activity pure water performs.

Some studies have shown that microwaving conserves more B vitamins (such as thiamin and riboflavin) and vitamin C than conventional cooking methods.

Vitamins and Minerals

We have noted the various vitamins and minerals that our bodies need. We need vitamins in very small amounts to regulate our body functions. There are two types of vitamins: water-soluble and fat-soluble. The body is able to store the fat-soluble vitamins for later use, but water-soluble vitamins need to be supplied continuously through the food we eat.

Minerals are essential for maintaining many body functions, ranging from building bones and teeth to keeping the heart and digestive system working smoothly. They are also required in very small amounts.

A comprehensive list of essential vitamins and minerals, their functions, food sources, and how much of each you need daily is found in the appendix.

To Supplement or Not to Supplement

It's not quite the question of the ages, but many women wonder if they need daily vitamin and mineral supplements. The answer? No, if your daily diet is balanced and adequate to your body's needs. Almost half of all Americans, however, do rely on daily supplements for the nutrition they should be getting from food. Probably this has something to do with the way supplements are advertised, promising longer, stronger, and better lives to all who will partake. One problem, though, many of these supplements are flushed through the body and offer no benefit at all. When they are improperly used they are not a good substitute for a well-balanced diet.

All that being said, in women at midlife, there may be a role for supplements. Particularly important is the need for calcium to protect your bones after menopause from the ravages of osteoporosis, which afflicts over 20 million people over the age of 45. You will want to talk to your doctor, pharmacist, or a registered dietitian, though, before you start taking anything. Consider having a thorough physical check-up and discuss your nutritional needs at that time.

When you do take supplements, be careful not to exceed the Recommended Dietary Allowances (RDA). Again, we've included the RDAs for essential vitamins and minerals in the appendix, page 229. Excess amounts of the water-soluble vitamins are excreted in the urine and so can do little damage, but the fat-soluble vitamins are stored in the body and may become toxic, so beware. The symptoms of toxicity for vitamin A, for example, include swelling of the ankles, loss of appetite and weight, fatigue, hair loss, throbbing headaches and vomiting, in extreme cases.

High-fiber diets provide protection against colon and rectal cancers and help bowel regularity. Whole wheat pasta packs about 6 grams of fiber in each 1/2 cup serving. Plus, it's fat free, high in complex carbohydrates, and rich in B vitamins, potassium, and iron.

Toxicity symptoms of vitamin D include appetite loss, diarrhea, dizziness, increased urination, muscle weakness, and weariness. When excessively high doses are consumed, you can also expect nausea, vomiting, and general weakness.

With vitamin E, you'll want to take special care. Vitamin E is often recommended for women during the perimenopause, just prior to the cessation of menses, and for a time after that. Vitamin E has been reported to be helpful for muscle cramps, but toxicity may result with excessive amounts. The tip-off that you're getting too much is elevated blood pressure.

If you don't make careful food choices and if your calorie intake is below what your body needs, you may want to consider taking a supplemental multi-vitamin/mineral. Several groups of women are more prone to deficiencies. These include women who are pregnant, the elderly, those on certain medications, finicky eaters, and heavy consumers of alcohol and/or tobacco products. If you are among these, talk to your doctor about which multiple supplement is right for you.

Attack of the Free Radicals

By now, nearly everyone has read a news article or two about the antioxidant vitamins and their possible role in slowing the aging process, reducing risks of heart disease and certain cancers, and combatting the effects of pollution. Some scientists studying the antioxidants believe that vitamins A, C, and E search out and destroy toxic molecules, known as "free radicals" that result from a specific process called oxidation. Unchecked, these free radicals are thought to damage artery walls and other healthy cells, and to contribute to the aging process.

Our attitude is that you should really plan your foodstyle so that you get as much of the antioxidant vitamins—A, C, and E—as you need from your food. If you are unable to do this, or if your doctor recommends that you take supplements, be sure you are aware of the potential toxicity of vitamins A and E. Be careful not to overdo the supplementation. There is still controversy as to how much of the water-solubles you retain, and there is clear evidence that fat-soluble vitamins can cause you harm.

Buyer Beware!

Many supplements are advertised as "natural" and claim to be superior to their synthetic counterparts. Vitamins are chemicals and the body can't determine whether they come from a plant, animal, or test tube.

The supplements found in your local grocery or drug store can be just as good (if not better) and are most definitely cheaper than their health food store counterparts. Plus you'll have a professional pharmacist available to you as well.

So, be sure to read labels, talk to the pharmacist, and if any product claims to provide you with more than just basic nutritional supplementation, beware! As a good rule of thumb, remember, if it sounds too good to be true, it probably is.

How Does Your Foodstyle Rate?

Before we continue, we invite you to take a few moments and rate your eating habits. It is a very telling way to see where you stand nutritionally. Just check the boxes on page 15 that most closely reflect your eating style, then add up your points according to the directions on page 16.

1.

a. ❑ *I eat 2 or more servings of fruit every day.*

b. ❑ *I eat 1 serving of fruit every day.*

c. ❑ *I rarely eat fruit, maybe an occasional banana or some grapes.*

2.

a. ❑ *I eat 3 or more servings of vegetables every day.*

b. ❑ *I eat 1 to 2 servings of vegetables every day.*

c. ❑ *I occasionally choose a tossed salad as a vegetable source with my meal.*

3.

a. ❑ *I eat 6 to 11 servings of whole grain breads, cereals, crackers, rice, or pasta every day.*

b. ❑ *I select whole grain products at least 3 to 5 times a week.*

c. ❑ *I typically eat 1 to 3 servings of bread, cereals, rice, or pasta, but prefer white over whole wheat.*

4.

a. ❑ *I eat 2 to 3 (2-3 ounce) servings of lean meat, poultry, fish, dried beans or tofu every day.*

b. ❑ *I select lean meat products at least 3 times a week.*

c. ❑ *I prefer to eat higher fat meats like chicken with skin or a thick steak, rather than skinless chicken breasts or fish.*

5.

a. ❑ *I eat 2 to 3 servings of low-fat or nonfat milk, yogurt, cheese, or dairy products every day.*

b. ❑ *I sometimes choose low-fat dairy products.*

c. ❑ *I prefer whole milk and regular ice cream instead of skim milk and frozen yogurt or sherbet.*

6.

a. ❑ *I exercise vigorously at least 3 times a week for a minimum of 30 minutes each time.*

b. ❑ *I exercise once or twice a week.*

c. ❑ *I occasionally take a long walk for exercise.*

Number of "a's"
checked _____ x 3 =_____

Number of "b's"
checked _____ x 2 =_____

Number of "c's"
checked _____ x 1 =_____

Total points _____

How do you rate?

15-18 points:
You have top-notch eating habits. You typically include a variety of choices in your daily diet. Keep up the good work.

11-14 points:
Your diet could use a little improvement. Aim to increase the variety in your daily diet and decrease any unnecessary fat.

10 or less:
You need help to select more nutritious choices. Seek variety by eating more fruits, vegetables, and whole grains and cut back on extra fat. A regularly scheduled exercise program would also be a good idea.

2
What Should You Eat?
Your Guide to Better Choices

W omen have been struggling for years to reduce the fat in their diets. But a reduced-fat diet alone isn't the answer. Ask anyone who lost 25 pounds and then gained 30 back. Sound familiar? We have found that many women cut fat out but then forget to increase their fiber intake. And what about upping fruits, vegetables, whole grains, dried beans and peas, as some diet programs recommend? How do we know if we are drinking enough milk? Do we get enough calcium to protect our aging bones? How about iron, how much do we need after menopause? How exactly can we tell if we're getting what we need? Just what is "eating right?"

The Great Pyramid

To answer some of these pressing questions, the U.S. Department of Agriculture has provided us with an illustrated food pyramid intended to guide us into making better dietary choices. As you review the pyramid in the following pages, notice the range of servings cited for each food group. The recommended number of servings is based on a variety of factors and includes your age, your sex, and your activity level. The lower number of servings is intended for children, older adults, and women. The higher number is for men, highly active women, and teenagers.

The Food Guide Pyramid is further intended for maintaining your weight. If you need to lose a few pounds, you'll want to read Chapter Three. For help in creating a personalized nutrition program that can accommodate your specific health needs, you may want to contact a registered dietitian who can provide you with an individualized program. (If you are unsure how to locate a registered dietitian, contact a local hospital or the National Center for Nutrition and Dietetics at 800-366-1655.)

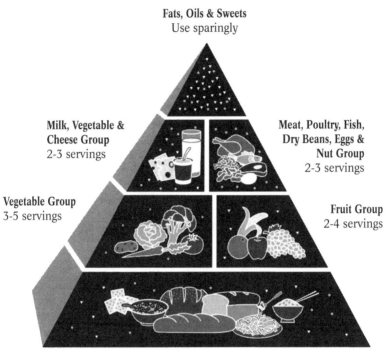

Fats, Oils & Sweets
Use sparingly

Milk, Vegetable &
Cheese Group
2-3 servings

Meat, Poultry, Fish,
Dry Beans, Eggs &
Nut Group
2-3 servings

Vegetable Group
3-5 servings

Fruit Group
2-4 servings

Bread, Cereal, Rice & Pasta Group
6-11 servings

The following chart adjusts the number of servings of each of the food groups by recommended daily calorie intake. These calorie recommendations are based on activity levels: less active women and most older adults need only 1600 calories to maintain their current weight; most children, teenage girls, active women, less active men, and some pregnant and lactating women need 2200 calories; most teenage boys, active men, and very active women need 2800 calories.

What Should You Eat?

They All Relate—Servings, Calories, Activities

Recommended number of servings adjusted for calorie intake and activity levels.

Food Group	Somewhat Active 1600 cal.	Very Active 2200 cal.	Highly Active 2800 cal.
Bread, cereal, rice, pasta	6	9	11
Fruits	2	3	4
Vegetables	3	4	5
Milk	2	2	2
Meat	2	2	3

To show you just how these servings can fit into your foodstyle, we have included a sample daily plan broken down into meals and snacks. We've used the 1600-calorie daily maintenance plan in this example. If you fit into a higher calorie category, add servings as needed. If you don't snack, fit those food choices into your mealtimes. Information follows about the types of foods in each group of the pyramid and sample serving sizes.

Sample 1600-Calorie Daily Food Plan

Breakfast—1 bread/starch, 1 fruit, 1 milk

example

1 bowl wheat flakes with sliced fresh peaches
1 cup of 2% milk

Lunch—1 meat, 2 bread/starch, 1 vegetable

example

Sliced smoked deli turkey on whole wheat kaiser roll with lettuce, tomato, sprouts, and Dijon mustard

Mid-afternoon snack—1 fruit

example

Fresh grapes

Dinner—1 meat, 2 bread/starch, 2 vegetables

example

Grilled pork tenderloin
Boiled parsley potato
Steamed broccoli
Apple/romaine/walnut salad

Evening snack—1 bread/starch, 1 milk

example

Teddy Grahams
Lite fruited yogurt

Small amounts of fat, oil, or salad dressings may be used, although no more than 3 servings or 3 teaspoons should be used daily. If more are desired, use nonfat or low-fat options (that is, nonfat salad dressings, light margarine, or light mayonnaise).

What Each Food Group on the Pyramid Contributes to the Daily Foodstyle

Let's begin at the base of the pyramid:

The bread group—

provides carbohydrates, B vitamins, and fiber. Good choices include whole grain breads and cereals, bagels, pita bread, English muffins, tortillas, breadsticks, pasta, rice, barley, couscous, pretzels, and popcorn. One serving is equal to:

- 1 slice of bread
- 1 ounce of dry cereal
- 1/2 of a bagel, English muffin, or hamburger bun
- 1 dinner roll, muffin, or tortilla
- 1/2 cup of rice, pasta or cooked cereal

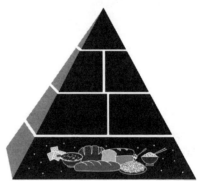

The fruit group—

contributes carbohydrates, vitamin A, vitamin C, and fiber. Good choices from this group include bananas, apples, oranges, grapefruit, plums, apricots, strawberries, grapes, cantaloupe, watermelon, mangoes, papayas, and fruit juice. A serving is equal to:

- 1 medium-sized fruit
- 3/4 cup fruit juice
- 1/2 cup canned fruit
- 1/4 small melon
- 1/4 cup dried fruit

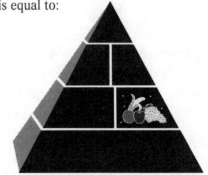

The vegetable group—

also provides carbohydrates, vitamins A and C, and fiber. Good choices include carrots, sweet potatoes, broccoli, brussel sprouts, cauliflower, peas, tomatoes, spinach, kale, squash, romaine lettuce, and vegetable juice. A serving is equal to:

- 1/2 cup vegetables, cut up
- 3/4 cup vegetable juice
- 1 medium-sized potato

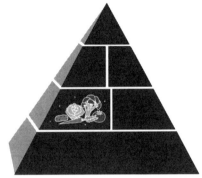

The milk group—

adds calcium, carbohydrates, protein, and vitamin D. Good choices include low-fat or nonfat milk, buttermilk, yogurt, cheese, and frozen yogurt. One serving is equal to:

- 1 cup milk or yogurt
- 1 1/2 ounces natural cheese
- 2 ounces processed cheese
- 1/2 cup ice cream, ice milk, or frozen yogurt

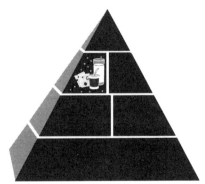

The meat group—

contributes primarily protein and iron. Good choices include skinless chicken, turkey, fish, eggs, lean meat, veal, dried beans (kidney, navy, black, pinto, and lentils), blackeyed peas, chick-peas, and split peas. A serving is equal to:

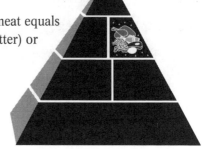

- 2 to 3 ounces lean meat,
  poultry, or fish (1 ounce of lean meat equals
  1 egg or 2 tablespoons peanut butter) or

- 1/2 cup cooked
  dry beans or peas

Do you wonder what makes a 3-ounce serving of meat? Well, one portion is just about the same size as a deck of cards. Here are some 3-ounce portions:

- 1 chicken breast
  (1 side of the chicken only)

- 4 ounces of raw meat
  (25% is lost when it is cooked)

- 3/4 cup tuna

- 3/4 cup chopped
  or ground meat

Have You Heard About 5-A-Day?

As a rule of thumb, think "5-A-Day" when it comes to meeting your quota of fruit and vegetable servings. It's an easy way to remember how many you should include in your personal foodstyle. Many women (and men, for that matter) tend to overlook the value of fruits and vegetables as snacks besides in meals. Fruits and vegetables are naturally low in fat, contain no cholesterol, are high in fiber, and add color and variety to meals. And, they're chock-full of nutrition! Of the 5-A-Day choices, be smart and opt for at least one high in vitamin A and one high in vitamin C. (See the appendix.)

At the tip of the pyramid, you'll find the extra, or bonus, foods—fats, oils, and sugar (this means salad dressings, soft drinks, and candy). These foods do not supply any particular nutrients, so try to limit their use. However, they do contribute calories and fat and should be included only if you need extra calories for energy.

Keep in mind the three key words:

balance - Select the appropriate number of servings each day.

variety - Make different choices within each group daily.

moderation - Select adequately sized portions and limit, don't eliminate, extra foods.

Of all the difficulties we face in life, our food choices and lifestyle tend to be our most challenging. Today, with the convenience of the microwave oven, take-out foods, and meal pick-ups or deliveries, we pay less attention to meal planning than ever before. Where once we planned each meal and did our grocery marketing regularly, we now tend to do what's easiest. And, if the frightening statistics on the incidence of cancer and heart disease tell us anything at all, they certainly suggest that the American diet is suffering as a result.

No one food or food group in the pyramid can supply all the nutrients you need for good health—it's the combination of all groups that covers all the bases.

Okay, we know that women have other responsibilities than just feeding themselves and their families. Life has changed. Food has changed. Cooking has changed. Organization is still the key, however, and with a little organization, you can get control over your foodstyle and work your way back to vibrant, young, and healthy living.

7 Steps to a Healthier Foodstyle

Here they are, in a nutshell:

1. Eat a variety of foods.

2. Watch calories and portion sizes.

3. Reduce fat and cholesterol.

4. Increase carbohydrates and high-fiber foods.

5. Use sugars in moderation.

6. Use salt and sodium in moderation.

7. If you drink alcoholic or caffeinated beverages, do so in moderation.

The Food Guide Pyramid places emphasis on healthy choices and selecting a variety of foods. It does not set rigid rules. Instead, it offers an eating outline that enables you to make better choices. Using this guide to select the appropriate types of food and the right number of servings will help you plan meals and daily menus that lead you to a foodstyle that can be both healthful and pleasurable.

1. Variety is the spice of life

Eating a wide variety of fruits, vegetables, whole grains, legumes, dairy products, meat, fish, and poultry is the foundation for a nutritious diet. Interestingly, most people tend to eat only about 10 to 20 foods and repeat these foods on a regular basis. Based on old habits and old taste memories, they are tied into a self-imposed food prison.

Well, here's one way to break out. Always include at least three different kinds of food at any given meal. Serve a bread, cereal, or pasta; include a fruit or vegetable or both; put in a dairy product and/or prepare some meat, poultry, fish, dried beans or peas, an egg, or even peanut butter.

Remember from Chapter 1, you need more than 50 different nutrients for good health, so meals consisting of just one food group (like a salad or a bowl of oatmeal) can't do the job. Take into consideration the pleasurable aspects of your dining experience. Try new tastes and textures.

2. Watch calories and portions

You've probably heard it said that "You can never be too rich or too thin."

Well, we can't comment on the "too rich" part, but the "too thin" part is simply not true. You can indeed be too thin, and being underweight can lead to serious problems as you grow older. For instance, some calorie reserves are necessary for periods of illness and body stress. Studies have shown that the uncomfortable symptoms of the perimenopause, like hot flashes and sleeplessness, are more troublesome to thinner women. But being over our desired weight can cause problems of another sort.

One cup of chopped, cooked broccoli supplies 90 percent of the daily requirement of beta carotene, 200 percent of the vitamin C, significant amounts of niacin, calcium, thiamin, and phosphorus, and 25 percent of your daily fiber needs.

Eating too much food isn't the only culprit behind weight gain. Lack of physical activity is a major player, too. Remember, food is simply fuel for the body. If you use more fuel in physical activity, you can take in more and still maintain a healthy weight. If you take in more fuel than you spend, you'll find yourself dealing with those "weighty" matters.

Also, we seem to need fewer calories as we age, since many of the calorie-consuming bodily activities, like growing, are complete. It is a smart idea to begin gradually lowering your caloric intake as soon as you notice that your levels of physical activity are lessening. For some women this is around age 35. The simple solution is to cut out bedtime snacks or refuse second servings. And here's where reducing fat in the diet can pay off. Fat measures in at twice the calories as protein or carbohydrates. So, the obvious conclusion: cut your fat intake. Detailed information on how to do this follows.

The good news is that cutting back on portion sizes and limiting second servings is often all most women need to do.

Here's a word to the wise: weight loss is temporary, but weight control lasts an entire lifetime.

3. Cut the fat and cholesterol

We've all read it. Newspaper headlines have reported it. Fat and cholesterol are our mortal enemies. Health professionals worldwide are urging all of us to lower our fat intake. Major health problems, namely heart disease and cancer, have been linked to the high-fat diet most Americans eat, as has obesity. The facts are that a diet high in saturated fat causes undesirable changes in the blood, increasing the level of LDL (the bad kind) of cholesterol.

Around 40 percent of the total daily caloric intake of most Americans is eaten as fat. The national goal: No more than 30 percent of all calories consumed should come from fat. Some health experts believe this number should be 25 percent. Remember, fat is found in meat, poultry, fish, eggs, milk, cheese, and other dairy products, in addition to the obvious sources such as oils, margarine, salad dressings, nuts, seeds, avocados, and butter.

Calories in Butter, Margarine, Oil, and Salad Dressings*

Food Product	Calories per Tbsp.
oil	135
butter	100
regular tub and stick margarine	100
spread tub and stick margarine	75
imitation diet margarine	50
mayonnaise	100
French dressing	85
Italian dressing	80
homemade oil and vinegar	70
Thousand Island dressing	60
mayonnaise-type dressing	58
Ranch dressing	54
reduced-calorie mayonnaise	50
reduced-calorie Thousand Island	25
reduced-calorie French	24
low-calorie Italian	5

*Exact calories may vary based on brand of food.

Fats are described as saturated or unsaturated. Saturated fats come mainly from animal sources, but sometimes you'll encounter them in cake mixes, crackers, cookies, nondairy products, or imitation whipped cream. Fruits, vegetables, and dried beans and peas (except for soybeans) contain very little fat. Plain breads and cereals are likewise very low in fat. With all this attention to the fat content in our diets, it is no wonder that many meat products are now available with reduced fat and dairy products are appearing daily sporting nonfat and low-fat labels.

Even though excess fat is bad for the body, our bodies still need some fat . . . albeit a small amount. So, don't cut fat out of your foodstyle altogether because in the long run, you'll do your body more harm than good. The essential fatty acids your body needs (linoleic and linolenic) come from fats, particularly oils, seeds, nuts, and wheat germ. By eliminating fat entirely, we deprive our bodies of these essential nutrients. Plus, there is nothing to "stick to your ribs" and you have to eat every 2 hours on very low-fat diets.

How Many Fat Calories per Day?

Daily Calories	Total Grams of Fat (30%)	Total Calories from Fat (9/gram)	Grams of Saturated Fat (10%)	Calories from Saturated Fat (30% of Total Fat)
1200	40	360	13	117
1500	50	450	17	153
1800	60	540	20	180
2000	67	600	22	198
2500	83	750	28	252
2700	90	810	30	270

Cutting back on cholesterol is not the same thing as cutting back on fat, even though both fat and cholesterol are often found in the same foods. Cholesterol, however, is found only in foods of animal origin, such as meat, fish, poultry, eggs, dairy products, and cheese. Organ meats and egg yolks are particularly high in cholesterol. And, in addition to what we get from food, in our bodies, the liver manufactures its own cholesterol.

> *Eating even small amounts of fish (a serving or two a week) can significantly reduce the risk of heart attack.*

Because cholesterol is very much like fat, it does not mix well with water. It is transported throughout the body in little packages called lipoproteins, which are made up of various amounts of cholesterol, triglycerides, and other proteins. There are two types of lipoproteins: high-density lipoprotein or HDL, and low-density lipoprotein or LDL. We remember these by associating the H in HDL with healthy and the L in LDL with lousy.

There is some scientific evidence that the HDL cholesterol benefits us by actually cleaning our arteries while the LDL seems to attract cholesterol and this cholesterol tends to accumulate in our arteries, causing clogging.

Cutting back on our intake of high-cholesterol foods definitely helps lower blood cholesterol levels, but lowering the amount of total fat and saturated fat we eat can actually yield a bigger benefit. For some people, however, medication must still be added to the mix of proper diet and activity levels to combat high blood cholesterol levels. Genetic factors are also at work here, so get advice from your doctor if your blood cholesterol levels are consistently high.

Typically, Americans have been known to consume 400 to 600 milligrams of cholesterol daily. That level is dropping with increased education about the dangers of high LDL. Today the recommended level is 300 milligrams or less. Three to four egg yolks a week, two daily servings of low-fat dairy products, or 6 to 7 ounces of meat a day can be worked into the 300-milligram guideline; it's a generous amount.

Saturated fat is much more the culprit in raising blood cholesterol levels than is consuming cholesterol itself in your diet. As you see from the following chart, saturated fat grams (13 grams is the goal for a 1200-calorie meal plan) add up quickly:

1 ounce cheddar cheese	6 grams of saturated fat
1 Tbsp. margarine	2.2 grams
3 ounces lean beef patty	6.2 grams
	14.4 grams of saturated fat

Just those three food items give you 1.4 grams more than your daily goal!

The table below lists the cholesterol and saturated fat content of some common foods we all like to include in our foodstyle. Take a look and use the table to help make better choices when you plan your meals.

Cholesterol and Saturated Fat Content of Common Foods

Food	Serving Size	Cholesterol (mg)	Saturated Fat (gm)
Milk, Cream			
milk, whole	1 cup	33	5
milk, skim	1 cup	4	0.3
cream, sour	1 Tbsp.	6	1.8
ice cream	1/2 cup	29	4.15
ice milk	1/2 cup	9	1.75
yogurt, plain low-fat	1/2 cup	7	1.13

Cholesterol and Saturated Fat Content of Common Foods, continued

Food	Serving Size	Cholesterol (mg)	Saturated Fat (gm)
Cheese			
cheddar	1 ounce	30	6
cottage, low-fat	1/2 cup	9	0.7
mozzarella	1 ounce	22	3.7
Swiss	1 ounce	26	5
Fats			
butter	1 Tbsp.	31	7.1
margarine	1 Tbsp.	0	2.2
corn oil	1 Tbsp.	0	1.7
olive oil	1 Tbsp.	0	1.8
peanut oil	1 Tbsp.	0	2.2
safflower oil	1 Tbsp.	0	1.2
soybean oil	1 Tbsp.	0	2
canola oil	1 Tbsp.	0	1
shortening	1 Tbsp.	0	3.3
mayonnaise	1 Tbsp.	8	1.7
Fruits, Vegetables	any amount	0	trace
Bread, Cereal	1 slice/oz.	0	trace
croissant	1	13	3.5

Cholesterol and Saturated Fat Content of Common Foods, continued

Food	Serving Size	Cholesterol (mg)	Saturated Fat (gm)
Desserts			
angel food cake	1 slice	0	.03
devil's food cake	1 slice	37	3.5
pound cake	1 slice	32	1.2
brownie	1 square	18	1.4
Grains, Pasta	any amount	0	trace
Meat, Fish, Poultry			
lean beef patty	3 oz.	74	6.2
lean pork	3 oz.	67	4
chicken breast (no skin)	3 oz.	73	0.87
flounder	3 oz.	58	0.3
salmon	3 oz.	74	1.6
shrimp	3 oz.	147	0.28
lobster claw	3 oz.	80	0.1
lobster tail	3 oz.	59	0.1
sardines	3 oz.	119	1.3
tuna (water pk)	3 oz.	48	0.14
liver, pork	3 oz.	302	1.2
frankfurter	1 (2 oz.)	27	6.8
egg	1	213	1.7

4. Increase your carbohydrates and high-fiber foods

There was a time when people believed that carbohydrates were responsible for making us fat. Well, that's simply not true. Carbohydrates are the body's preferred nutrient—the best source of energy. They are also the easiest and quickest food to digest. Carbohydrates are divided into two general categories: starches and fibers, known as complex carbohydrates, and sugars, referred to as simple carbohydrates.

Grain products, bread, and starchy vegetables such as potatoes, dried beans, and peas are all rich in complex carbohydrates. The advantage of these foods is that they are digested relatively slowly and contain fiber. Fiber helps us to feel full, so fiber foods go a long way when it comes to weight control.

Fiber is actually the part of the plant that our bodies cannot digest, but it still plays a major role in the health of the human digestive tract. There are six fiber components found in foods: cellulose, hemicellulose, lignin, pectin, mucilage, and gums. Not every high-fiber food has all six of these components, nor does each component have the same effect on the body. The fiber in food is actually measured by taking a measurement of the amount of fiber that is left after the body has digested the food. The residue, called dietary fiber, is measured in grams and is currently listed on food labels.

For high fiber foods eat bran, whole grains, oats, legumes, dried beans and peas, barley, and fresh fruits and vegetables.

Dietary fiber is also categorized as either soluble or insoluble, according to its solubility in water. Insoluble fiber contains lignin, cellulose, and some hemicellulose, and it does not dissolve in water. Thus it cannot be digested and it tends to speed up the rate at which food passes through the intestines, taking along with it any potentially harmful substances and wastes.

Insoluble fiber is the "roughage" our grandmothers talked about. It is an important part of any diet and there is evidence that it may help reduce the risk of colon cancer. Insoluble fiber is found in wheat bran, whole grains, fruits, vegetables, and some varieties of nuts.

Soluble fiber contains pectin, gum, mucilage, and some hemicellulose. It does, as the name suggests, dissolve in water. It is found in oats, dried beans and peas, barley, and some fruits such as oranges and apples. Soluble fiber is thought to absorb substances that the body uses to make cholesterol, removing them from the body via the gastrointestinal tract. Theoretically, this would suggest that it reduces cholesterol levels in the blood.

It has also been suggested that soluble fiber helps to improve blood sugar levels but only when eaten in very large amounts. (More oatmeal than you'd want to eat!)

There actually are plenty of good reasons to increase the amount of high-fiber foods in your foodstyle. A high-fiber diet can help prevent constipation and can reduce the incidence of gastrointestinal tract problems like appendicitis, polyps, colitis, diverticulosis, and even large bowel and rectum cancers.

How fiber works exactly is not yet firmly established. It appears, however, to be closely linked to the length of time food stays in the large intestine and to the amount of bacteria in the colon. If fiber pushes food through the intestine, less bacteria act on the colon, potentially reducing future health problems with the colon.

Currently, the average person eats only about 11 grams of dietary fiber daily. For good health, we recommend 20 to 30 grams of fiber every day. Here's a chart of the fiber content of a variety of common foods to help you schedule the "right stuff" into your personal foodstyle plan.

Looking for Fiber in All the Right Places

Fiber Content of Common Foods

Food	Serving Size	Grams of Dietary Fiber
Breads		
bran muffin	1 medium	3
oatbran muffin	1 medium	1.5
pumpernickel bread	1 slice	1
rye bread	1 slice	1
saltine crackers	4 crackers	0
white bread	1 slice	1
whole wheat bread	1 slice	2
Vegetables		
beans, kidney, cooked	1/2 cup	7
beans, pinto, cooked	1/2 cup	10
broccoli, cooked	1/2 cup	3
cabbage, raw	1/2 cup	2
carrots, cooked	1/2 cup	3
celery	1 stalk	less than 1
corn	1/2 cup	3
cucumber	6 slices	less than 1
green beans, cooked	1/2 cup	2
green pepper	2 slices	less than 1

Food	Serving Size	Grams of Dietary Fiber
Vegetables (continued)		
lettuce	1/2 cup	1
peas, cooked	1/2 cup	4
potato, baked with skin	1	4
potato, mashed	1/2 cup	1
potato, french fries	10 fries	1
potato, sweet	1/2 medium	2
tomato	1/2	1
Cereals and Pasta		
barley, pearled, uncooked	1/3 cup	9
bran cereal	1 ounce	8
bran flakes	1 ounce	4
brown rice	1/2 cup	less than 1
corn flakes	1 ounce	less than 1
oat bran	1 ounce	4
oatmeal	1 ounce	2
popcorn	1 cup	2
raisin bran	1 ounce	4
spaghetti	1 cup	2
spaghetti, whole wheat	1 cup	4.5
white rice	1/2 cup	less than 1

Fiber Content of Common Foods, continued

Food	Serving Size	Grams of Dietary Fiber
Fruits and Nuts		
apricot	1 medium	1
almonds	1/4 cup	5
apple	1 medium	3
banana	1 medium	3
cantaloupe	1/4 cup	2
grapefruit	1/2	1
orange	1 medium	2
peach	1 medium	3
peanut butter	2 tablespoons	2
peanuts	1/4 cup	3
pineapple	1/2 cup	1
prunes	1/3 cup	1.5
raisins	2 tablespoons	1
strawberries	1 cup	3

"Absorb" More Soluble Fiber

Food	Serving Size	Soluble Fiber (grams)	Total Grams of Dietary Fiber
apple with skin	1	1	3
baked potato	1	2	4
blackeyed peas	1/2 cup	3.7	10
corn	1/2 cup	1.5	3
figs	5	5	9
green peas	1/2 cup	2	4
kidney beans	1/2 cup	3	7
oat bran cereal, cooked	1/2 cup	2	4
oatmeal	3/4 cup	1.4	3
prunes	1/3 cup	1.5	3
split peas, cooked	1/2 cup	1.5	5

5. Use the sweet stuff in moderation

Okay, so what about sugar? Most of us think that sugar is that white granulated stuff we add to coffee and put in baked goods. But, actually, there are many different kinds of sugar. They can be divided into two groups: those that occur naturally in foods (such as fruits, vegetables, and milk), and those that are added during food processing or to foods at home.

Although sugars enter your body in different forms, all are converted to glucose or blood sugar within 1 to 1 1/2 hours. In reality, your body can't distinguish where the sugar came from originally, it only knows it's there.

Sugar has been blamed for causing diabetes, obesity, hyperactivity, and heart disease, but only dental caries (tooth decay) are actually caused directly by sugar. Eating sugar does not cause diabetes. Rather, diabetes is a disease characterized by the body's inability to use sugar properly. Thus, high blood sugar or high glucose levels are the identifying symptoms of diabetes.

Questions about nutrition? Contact the National Center for Nutrition and Dietetics at (800) 366-1655.

Eating sugar does not cause obesity, either. But, many foods high in sugar are also high in fat and calories, and these can cause obesity. High sugar intakes were once associated with antisocial, aggressive, or criminal behaviors, but when studied, no direct correlation was ever found.

Finally, no conclusive evidence exists to date that links sugar directly to risk factors for heart disease. Again, diets high in sugar are usually likewise high in fat and calories and short on vitamins, minerals, and fiber. Not surprisingly, a high-fat diet is strongly implicated in heart disease.

The average American today derives 24 percent of all daily calories from sugar. This is too high. The recommendation is to reduce this level to not more than 10 percent. This means that on a 2,000 calorie daily plan, you can still have a light dessert, but you need to be aware of the sugar content of processed foods, so read labels. When we do eat sugar, our goal should be to get it in its natural state, as from milk, fruits, and vegetables.

Sugar Aliases

Carefully read food labels and be aware that sugar has lots of names, such as:

—honey   —brown sugar
—invert sugar   —confectioner's sugar
—maple sugar   —corn sweeteners

- —molasses
- —raw sugar
- —turbinado sugar
- —sucrose
- —high fructose corn syrup or HFCS

- —corn syrup
- —dextrose
- —fructose
- —granulated sugar

What about artificial sweeteners?

Every day millions of women use artificial sweeteners, thinking to avoid the extra calories of too much sugar. Saccharin, for example, was discovered a century ago and has been used as a noncaloric sweetener in foods and beverages for over 80 years. In fact, in the 1970s, it was the only low-calorie sweetener in use.

Since the '70s, other new low-calorie sweeteners have been approved by the Food and Drug Administration (FDA), and include aspartame and acesulfame K. Some foods contain other sweeteners such as fructose and the sugar alcohols—sorbitol, mannitol, maltitol, and xylitol. These, however, contain as many calories as regular sugar and should not be used if your goal is weight control.

The FDA has established acceptable daily intakes (ADIs) for both aspartame and acesulfame K. The ADI is the amount a person can safely consume on a daily basis (over the span of a lifetime) without adverse effect. A 100-fold safety factor is built into the ADI by the FDA.

Hop on the "bran" wagon by starting your day with a high fiber cereal or bran muffin.

Saccharin is considered safe for human consumption, but there has been some controversy over the appropriate levels in which it remains safe. In 1977, the U.S. Congress passed a moratorium preventing the FDA from banning saccharin altogether in the U.S. This moratorium is in effect until 1997, so saccharin remains available on the American market.

Artificial sweeteners, in general, when used in reasonable amounts, seem to pose no health risks for most people. For vibrant, young, healthy living, however, their use should be moderate, particularly for pregnant women.

Here's the skinny on artificial sweeteners.

Acesulfame K (known as Sunette® or Sweet One®):

- is 200 times more sweet than granulated sugar.
- contains no calories.
- leaves no aftertaste.
- is not metabolized by the body.
- can be used in cooking and baking.

Aspartame (known as Nutrasweet® or Equal®):

- is 180 times more sweet than granulated sugar.
- contains very few calories.
- leaves no aftertaste.
- tastes very much like granulated sugar.
- contains two amino acids that are metabolized by the body.
- cannot be used in baking (high heat).
- is considered safe in pregnancy.
- must be restricted in children and adults with phenylketonuria (PKU).

Cyclamates:

- are 30 to 60 times more sweet than sugar.
- were removed from the FDA's "Generally Recognized as Safe" (GRAS) list in 1969.

Saccharin (known as Sweet 'n Low®, Sprinkle Sweet®, or Sugar Twin®):

- is calorie free.

- leaves a bitter aftertaste when consumed in large amounts.

- can be used in baking.

- is not metabolized by the body.

- not recommended for use during pregnancy.

The following are known as nutritive sweeteners and contain calories.

Sugar alcohols, made from sorbitol, mannitol, maltitol, or xylitol:

- are absorbed in the body as carbohydrates, but very slowly.

- do not promote tooth decay.

- have the same number of calories as sugar (4 calories/gram), although they are labeled sugar-free.

- are 50 to 100 percent as sweet as granulated sugar.

- can cause diarrhea if used in excess.

- usually found in higher fat desserts.

Fructose:

- is the sweetest of all the sugars.

- may increase cholesterol levels at high intakes (more than 20% of the total daily calories).

- are fruit sugars (from honey or fruits).

- contain a monosaccharide such as glucose.

- have the same number of calories as granulated sugar.

- is converted to glucose (blood sugar) in the liver.

- offer no metabolic advantages over granulated sugar.

6. Use salt and sodium in moderation

Salt is a combination of two minerals, sodium and chloride. We need both minerals to survive since they are the principle regulators of the water balance in our body fluids and our cells. Too much salt has been implicated in hypertension, particularly in people who have a family history of high blood pressure.

Chill soups, stews, broths, and sauces in the refrigerator. The fat will rise to the top and harden to be lifted off.

If untreated, hypertension can lead to strokes, heart attacks, and kidney disease, so health experts recommend moderation in our intake of sodium. Today, the recommended sodium intake level is 2,400 to 3,000 milligrams or less, although some controversy exists about salt-restricted diets. One teaspoon of salt contains 2,000 milligrams of sodium.

Salt is probably THE leading additive, both in processed foods and at the dining table. But the truth is that there is enough sodium naturally present in the foods we eat and in our water supply to more than meet our daily needs. People who work or exercise in very hot weather and lose a lot of fluids through perspiration need to replace those fluids by drinking lots of water.

Sodium Aliases

Watch food labels for hidden sources of sodium, which is listed as:

—monosodium glutamate or MSG
—disodium phosphate
—sodium bicarbonate (baking soda)
—sodium aluminum sulfate (baking powder)
—sodium benzoate

—salt

The following list indicates the sodium content of some basic foods likely to be part of an average foodstyle:

Salt of the Earth

Item	Serving Size	Mg. of Sodium
Protein Foods		
corned beef	4 oz.	1474
tuna, water packed with salt	3.5 oz.	866
lasagna	1 piece	760
ham	2 oz.	746
cheese pizza	1/8 of 15" pie	699
frankfurter	2 oz.	627
scallops	4 oz.	300
bacon	2 slices	153
peanut butter	1 Tbsp.	97
hamburger	4 oz.	82
round steak	4 oz.	80
egg	1 large	61
chicken, dark meat	4 oz.	60
chicken, light meat	4 oz.	45
tuna, water packed no salt	3.5 oz.	41

Sodium Content, continued

Item	Serving Size	Mg. of Sodium
Dairy Products		
American cheese	1 oz.	322
buttermilk	8 oz.	319
cottage cheese	4 oz.	241
processed cheese spread	1 Tbsp.	228
cheddar cheese	1 oz.	199
low-fat milk	8 oz.	150
yogurt	8 oz.	125
ice cream	8 oz.	84
Bread, Pasta, Cereals		
saltine crackers	10	312
corn flakes	1 cup	251
white bread	1 slice	122
whole wheat bread	1 slice	121
noodles	1 cup	3
rice	1 cup	trace
puffed rice cereal	1 cup	trace
Fruits and Vegetables		
sauerkraut	1/2 cup	560
green beans, canned	1/2 cup	302

Sodium Content, continued

Item	Serving Size	Mg. of Sodium
Fruits and Vegetables (continued)		
corn, canned	1/2 cup	266
lima beans, frozen	1/2 cup	86
celery	1/2 cup	75
broccoli	1/2 cup	50
carrots	1/2 cup	45
cantaloupe	1 wedge	19
pineapple	2/3 cup	7
grapes	1 cup	5
green beans, fresh	1/2 cup	3
orange	1	2
strawberries	1 cup	1
lima beans	1/2 cup	1
corn, fresh	1/2 cup	trace
Fats and Oils		
Italian dressing	1 Tbsp.	314
green olive	1	150
margarine	1 Tbsp.	140
Thousand Island dressing	1 Tbsp.	112
mayonnaise	1 Tbsp.	84
black olive	1	75
oil	1 Tbsp.	0

Item	Serving Size	Mg. of Sodium
Other		
salt	1 Tbsp.	6589
canned soup	1/2 can	1500
soy sauce	1 Tbsp.	1379
dill pickle	medium	928
peach pie	1 slice	423
baking powder	1 tsp.	402
almonds, salted	1/2 cup	156
catsup	1 Tbsp.	156
mustard	1 tsp.	63

Pass the salt substitute, please

There are quite a few salt substitutes available, but you should get a recommendation from your physician before you start using one of them.
Many are made from potassium chloride and may affect your heart or
interfere with medications. Lots of the "light salts" are actually half regular salt and are really not salt-free. Sea salt, too, is still salt.

There are also many herbs and spices that you can use to season food in
place of salt. Look for salt-free herb mixes at the grocer. Many can be
used as a salt replacement at the table, as can pepper and lemon wedges.

Many of us are confused about what spices to use with which foods. The
following chart provides a guide. Actually, the options are endless, so
experiment to find out what complements your personal foodstyle.

Salt Shaker Replacements

Food Item	Try these Seasonings
beef	bay leaf, green pepper, fresh mushrooms, onion, pepper, sage, thyme
chicken	green pepper, lemon juice, paprika, sage, thyme, parsley, marjoram
fish	bay leaf, curry powder, lemon juice, marjoram, fresh mushrooms, paprika
pork	apple, garlic, onion, sage
asparagus	mustard seed, sesame seed, tarragon, lemon juice, garlic, onion, vinegar
broccoli	caraway seed, mustard seed, dill, tarragon
cabbage	caraway seed, celery seed, dill, mint, nutmeg, savory
carrots	allspice, bay leaf, dill, fennel, ginger, marjoram, nutmeg, mint
cauliflower	caraway seed, dill, tarragon
corn	green pepper, cayenne pepper, pimento, fresh tomato, chili powder
cucumbers	chives, dill, garlic, vinegar
green beans	dill, lemon juice, marjoram, pimento
peas	basil, mint, fresh mushrooms, onion, parsley
potatoes	green pepper, mace, onion, paprika, parsley, chives
rice	chives, green pepper, onion, saffron
spinach	basil, mace, marjoram, nutmeg, oregano

Salt Shaker Replacements, continued

Food Item	Try these Seasonings
squash	allspice, brown sugar, cinnamon, cloves, ginger, mace, nutmeg, rosemary, onion
tomatoes	basil, marjoram, onion, oregano, tarragon, thyme

Tips for herbs and spices:

• Use only a small amount; they are concentrated.

• Spices lose their flavor during cooking, so add them at the end of preparation.

• Store spices away from heat. Try them fresh. Grow your own, if you like.

7. If you drink alcoholic or caffeinated beverages, do so in moderation

Hippocrates, the "Father of Medicine," proclaimed wine "a nourishing beverage, a cooling agent against fevers, a dressing for wounds, a purgative, and a diuretic." And, you know, he was right. Moderate use of alcohol is not harmful for most people.

Today we recognize that many women have less tolerance to alcohol than men. But why? Women seem to feel the effects of alcohol faster because we are generally smaller than men and have less body fluid. It also takes longer for alcohol to leave the female body, new studies show, because women have lower levels of dehydrogenase, an enzyme that breaks down alcohol. Hormone fluctuations the week before menstruation also increase the effects of alcohol.

Yes, a glass of wine or an alcoholic drink can relieve tension, create a sense of well-being, and stimulate the appetite. But, we know that drinking too much can lead to many health problems. Heavy drinking is associated with cancers of the mouth, throat, esophagus, and liver. And, if you mix cigarette smoking with drinking, the risk of cancer increases even more. Besides being high in calories, alcohol is lacking in almost all vitamins and minerals.

So, just what is moderate drinking? Well, today's experts say that one to two drinks per day is enough for anyone.

Just what is a drink?

One drink might mean different things to each of us, so here's how we figure the amount of alcohol that equals a "drink."

—1 ounce 80 proof distilled spirits
  (70 calories)

—12 ounces regular beer (150 calories)

—12 ounces light beer (90 calories)

—4 ounces wine (80 calories)

—2 ounces sherry (75 calories)

Don't be fooled by literature that encourages the use of alcohol to reduce your risk of heart disease. Read what the scientific studies have shown, and remember, moderation is the key. A direct correlation between the use of alcohol and the incidence of breast cancer has recently been found, so talk to your doctor if you have any questions about your intake of alcohol.

Caffeine: moderation again

The jury is not in yet on what's the safest recommendation for use of caffeine. And, the research is often confusing. Here are some facts, but you need to decide what's best for you. After all, nobody knows your body better than you do.

Caffeine acts as a stimulant to the central nervous system. So, it is true that coffee, tea, and caffeine-laden cola drinks give you a lift. Caffeine helps you stay awake and alert, dilates certain blood vessels and constricts others, and increases your capacity to do muscular work and exercise. It is also a diuretic.

Some women are more sensitive to caffeine and react to it more intensely than others. A woman who doesn't drink coffee regularly will feel the effects of one cup more strongly than a woman who normally drinks several cups a day. Excessive consumption can lead to the "coffee jitters," anxiety, restlessness, inability to sleep, diarrhea, headaches, heart palpitations, stomach ulcers, and irregular heart beat.

Brown meats by broiling or sauteeing in a hot, nonstick pan, sprayed with vegetable cooking spray only if needed. If you use oil, pour it into a measuring spoon and then into the pan to avoid using too much. Each teaspoon of oil contains 45 calories and 5 grams of fat.

At one time it was thought that caffeinism was the most prominent disorder among Americans. Some women, when they attempt to curtail coffee consumption, will experience actual withdrawal symptoms: headaches, irritability, fatigue, and restlessness.

So, how much is too much? Some experts today recommend limiting coffee to one or two cups a day. For most women, moderate caffeine consumption in the range of 200 to 300 milligrams daily seems safe. But, if you are prone to feeling nervous, have stomach ulcers, or experience irregular heart beats, you should probably avoid caffeine as much as possible. During pregnancy and lactation, most experts agree that caffeine should be avoided, or limited to only one cup a day.

Caffeine is found in coffee and cocoa beans (chocolate), cola nuts, and tea leaves. Coffee, tea, and cola beverages are the three most popular beverages around the world.

The amount of caffeine in a beverage depends on many factors:

- The variety of coffee bean or tea leaf and where it is grown

- The grind of coffee or cut of tea leaf (the finer the grind, the more caffeine)

- The method of brewing (drip coffee has more caffeine than perked or instant)

- The length of brewing (the longer it's steeped, the more caffeine it contains)

The caffeine content of cocoa beans varies, but the caffeine in soft drinks is standardized. About 90 percent of the caffeine in cola beverages is added by the manufacturer. Today many colas are available without added caffeine.

3 easy ways to add fruit to you life: add it to lettuce salads, rice and stuffings, and low-fat yogurt.

In many areas, trendy coffee shops have sprung up, attracting women by offering a quick cup of flavored coffee, cappuccino, or espresso. These beverages also contain caffeine and should be consumed only in moderation. Although flavored coffees without added cream or sugar contain very few, if any, calories, some speciality coffee drinks can add more than 250 calories to your diet, causing weight gain over time. Many of these coffeehouses can make cappuccinos, lattes, and mochas with skim milk, which actually foams better. They also come decaffeinated. So how about ordering a decaf cappuccino with skim milk when you are tempted to stop for a cup?

One final note about caffeine: many prescription drugs contain caffeine, so read labels and know what you are taking. The following chart shows some of the common sources of caffeine and their caffeine content.

Where Lurks the Caffeine?

Food/Drink/ Drug	Serving Size	Mg. Caffeine
Coffee		
Instant	5 oz.	57
Perked	5 oz.	103
Dripped	5 oz.	151
Decaffeinated	5 oz.	2
Tea, black		
5-minute brew	5 oz.	46
1-minute brew	5 oz.	28
Hot cocoa	5 oz.	8
Colas and caffeine-containing carbonated beverages		
Low calorie or regular	12 oz.	36 to 52
Nonprescription drugs		
Headache remedies and pain relievers	1 tablet	32 to 60

Where lurks the caffeine, continued

Food/Drink/ Drug	Serving Size	Mg. Caffeine
Nonprescription drugs (continued)		
Cold preparations	1 tablet	about 30
Stimulants	1 tablet	about 100
Prescription drugs		
Depending on drug (talk to your doctor)	1 tablet	30 to 100

Remember, caffeine-free carbonated beverages and non-colas are available. However, there is some evidence that decaffeinated beverages should also be used in moderation. Reports on the safety of the various solvents and processes used to decaffeinate beverages have opened a Pandora's box of questions about this. When in doubt, talk to your doctor or your registered dietitian.

3

Weighing the Odds:

Losing & Winning
with Weight Control

More than half the women in the United States consider themselves overweight. And almost half of these are trying to lose weight at any given time. Dieting seems to be a national obsession for American women. It seems many are more concerned with losing pounds than with being healthy. When the weight obsession meets the youth obsession at midlife, the problems can seem overwhelming.

The American population overall is gaining more weight each year, tipping the scales higher than they should as a whole. This is despite the fact that many of us are dieting to lose. Part of the reason for this paradox is the lack of healthy eating habits in general; another reason is our national trend toward physical inactivity.

As we continue to gain weight at rates exceeding those of our ancestors, American women continue to look for quick, easy, and painless ways to lose weight. Billions of dollars are spent each year on various weight-loss programs, books, tapes, equipment, and diet foods. Women feel pressured into dropping pounds, often for the wrong reasons.

It is a fact that as we age our bodies change, our hormone levels change, our lifestyles change, and we change. It's not unlikely at midlife that you suddenly realize you've gained weight. Twenty or thirty pounds of weight gain doesn't really happen overnight, however. It's usually the case that you've added one or two pounds a year for 10 or 20 years.

Also, there's the weight gain that is associated with the perimenopause, the years just before your periods stop. Many women find that they are gaining weight during these years despite increasing their physical activity and restricting their diets. While this doesn't happen for all women, and while the mechanism that predisposes some women to gain weight during these years remains a mystery, to those women who fret over those extra pounds, we say, "Give yourself a break!" It's okay to have a few extra pounds during the menopausal years. If you are overly concerned about this, however, discuss it in detail with your doctor. A 14-year study completed recently did find that women who gained 11 to 18 pounds after age 18 had a 25 percent greater chance of suffering or dying of a heart attack than women who gained less than 11 pounds.

The fact is we simply need fewer calories to maintain a desirable weight as we get older. The percentage of muscle in our bodies decreases and the percentage of fat increases. When we become less active, we can lose up to half a pound of muscle a year. With less muscle, metabolism in the body slows down. Because fat tissue uses less energy than muscle tissue, a body with a higher proportion of fat needs fewer calories to maintain the same weight.

For boneless raw meat, fish, or chicken, buy 4-ounce portions. Count on shrinkage of about 25 percent in cooking. You'll end up with a 3-ounce portion, the size of a deck of cards. That's just the right size for most women.

If, for example, at age 20 you needed 2200 calories to maintain your weight, you may need only 1900 to maintain that same weight at age 45. The number of calories needed continues to decline as you get older. Calorie needs, as a matter of fact, drop about 10 percent for each decade we live beyond age 40. Unfortunately, many of us continue to eat the same amounts and kinds of food we always have and become less active, and this is what leads to weight gain.

Are you an Apple or Pear?

As women get older and accumulate some extra weight, where the weight settles can make a difference to overall health. The "pear-shape" body, with weight stored in the hips and thighs, is actually more desirable than the "apple-shape" body, where excess weight is distributed around one's middle, where the vital organs are located. Excess weight here adds to our risk of heart disease, diabetes, high blood pressure, and certain types of cancer.

Unfortunately, our shape is something beyond our control; it's been programmed into our genes. But, if you are predisposed to be an "apple," there are things you can do to reduce your risks. "Apple" shapes may want to consider losing weight for health reasons. "Pear" shapes, on the other hand, seem to want to lose weight for reasons of vanity. The fact is, too much weight on any shape body is not healthy for anyone of us.

What Should You Weigh?

Weight charts pop up periodically with varying weights for different age groups. Each person is different, and it's not easy to put an exact number on any given individual. Age, sex, body size, bone structure, genetics, fat-muscle ratio, and other factors all contribute to different weights for different people. It's possible that you might fit into a standard weight chart but still have too much body fat.

On the other hand, you may have more muscle than fat, look very lean, and yet be off the chart in terms of weight. This is because muscle weighs more than fat. The only way to know for sure how your fat-muscle ratio fits into the overall picture is to opt for tests that require weighing underwater or use of bioelectric devices that use electrical impulses to determine your percentage of body fat.

Trim as much fat as you can from meat before you freeze it or before you cook it. Also, remove all skin and visible fat from chicken. Good news: fish has no fat to trim!

Some health professionals can give you an idea of your body composition, that is the fat-to-muscle ratio, by using skinfold calipers, a less-expensive method of measurement. This is not as accurate as other tests, however. A desirable amount of body fat for a slim woman ranges between 18 and 22 percent. Body fat should not be less than 16 percent on any woman, nor should it be more than 30 percent.

The weight chart on the next page provides a range of weight at each height to allow for the variations that must be taken into account. Weight charts only measure total weight, not the difference between fat and muscle. Not everyone will fit into this chart. And, actually, it may be better to be heavier than your ideal weight throughout your life than to "yo-yo" up and down to fit into the chart.

Some people always seem to be dieting. One year they're down 30 pounds, but the next year they are up 40. And this cycle continues. This kind of dieting can cause more harm to your body than if you just keep the extra weight on in the first place.

Osteoporosis is preventable: Get plenty of calcium and vitamin D and do more weight-bearing activities such as running, tennis, low-impact aerobics, and walking.

The more you diet, the more body muscle you lose. This causes the metabolism to slow down. When weight is regained, more body fat is added, thus it becomes harder and harder to lose the excess pounds on the next diet. The cycle becomes frustrating and dangerous for your body.

It doesn't make any sense to diet if it's only going to be temporary and the weight you lose will be back again next year. To make sure the weight stays off for good, you need to change your eating habits and add exercise to your lifestyle.

Women today, especially young women, seemed programmed to want to look like models, movie stars, or beauty queens. As a result, we have an obsession with weight control and an epidemic of eating disorders. Don't get hung up on numbers on the bathroom scale. The weight chart is just a guide. If you feel good, look good, eat healthfully, and exercise regularly, enjoy life the way you are. Don't force yourself to be something you're not.

Fitting In*

| Height | Weight (in pounds) | |
	Ages 35 and Over	Ages 19 to 34
5'0"	108-138	97-128
5'1"	111-143	101-132
5'2"	115-148	104-137
5'3"	119-152	107-141
5'4"	122-157	111-146
5'5"	126-162	114-150
5'6"	130-167	118-155
5'7"	134-172	121-160
5'8"	138-178	125-164
5'9"	142-183	129-169
5'10"	146-188	132-174
5'11"	151-194	136-179
6'0"	155-199	140-184
6'1"	159-205	144-189
6'2"	164-210	148-195

(Measurements without clothes and shoes)

Source: U.S. Dept. of Agriculture, U.S. Dept. of Health and Human Services, Dietary Guidelines for Americans, 1990.

*Other, more technical ways to determine if you are underweight, overweight, or at a reasonable weight are to calculate you body mass index and waist-to-hip ratio.

Calculating Your Calories

Use this simple formula to determine the number of daily calories it takes to maintain your current weight. The formula gives you a "ballpark" figure and will vary from woman to woman, depending on your level of activity, the amount of muscle versus fat in your body, and your age.

Multiply your current weight in pounds (_____) by :

> 10 if you are inactive
>
> 12 if you are moderately active
>
> 15 if you are extremely active

This number equals the calories needed for the day to maintain your current weight.   (_____)

Now, let's try the formula again using your desired weight.

Multiply your desired weight in pounds (_____) by:

> 10 if you are inactive
>
> 12 if you are moderately active
>
> 15 if you are extremely active

This equals the number of calories you need for the day to maintain your desired weight. (_____)

Strive to eat the number of calories allowed for your desired weight, if you want to achieve that weight. This formula, even though simple, does take into account weight, activity levels, and the required energy to sustain them.

Calories Do Count

When making pot roast, trim all visible fat. Some recipes call for two tablespoons of fat for browning—that's 250-plus calories of extra fat. You can brown with one teaspoon fat in a nonstick pan and pour off the extra fat that comes from the meat. Just add water and flour to make gravy. Making all of these changes could save more than 300 calories and 30 grams of fat per serving.

First of all, to understand more about the contribution of calories you should know what a calorie is. Stated simply, a calorie measures energy supplied by food.

Calories (or food energy) basically come from three food sources, as we said in Chapter 1. The food sources are protein, carbohydrates, and fat—plus alcohol, which we don't consider a food source. Protein and carbohydrates each contribute 4 calories per gram of food. Fat contributes 9 calories per gram. You may get tired of reading this, but this fact explains why it's better to consume most of your calories from protein or carbohydrates instead of from fat. Alcohol, by the way, contributes 7 calories per gram and, as we said, is not a food source.

Furthermore, dietary fat is more easily converted to body fat than are protein and carbohydrates. Fat makes fat easily, whereas it takes about 23 percent more energy to convert carbohydrates and protein to fat.

Today when we shop, we are bombarded with nonfat, fat-free, and low-fat foods that appeal to fat-conscious consumers. Women, in particular, are seemingly going wild over these products, especially those foods that have always been taboo on a weight-reduction diet.

What many people don't realize, however, is that these foods still contain calories from the other energy-producing nutrients. Many of them are high in sugar to compensate for the flavor lost when fat is eliminated. Others are extremely high in salt. While low-fat and fat-free products are fine, when used in moderation, if consumed in excess, they will cause weight gain! Beyond this, they are expensive, too.

It is far better to turn to foods that are naturally low in fat. Plus, they will be easy on your pocketbook. One study, as reported in *Health* magazine, determined a family of four could save more than $1,500 a year by using a few "smart" grocery shopping techniques. The Research Institute at Bassett Health Care, in Cooperstown, New York, tracked 291 people after adopting a 30-percent-calories-from-fat diet. Three months into the healthier diet, people most closely following the advice were saving $5 a week. At nine months, after getting the hang of it, they were shaving $8 a week off their grocery bill. Some suggestions include:

> *Don't let "no cholesterol" margarine labels fool you. It's the fat and calorie content that's important. Besides, all margarine is cholesterol-free. Only real butter contains cholesterol.*

- *Cut back on meat.* Burgers for a family of four require two pounds of ground beef ($4), buns (50 cents), and some lettuce, tomatoes, and onions ($1.75), for a total of $6.25. Not bad, but take the beef for one burger ($1) and mix it with tomato paste, onion, mushrooms, garlic, and bay leaf ($1.25) for spaghetti sauce, serve it over noodles ($1), and the cost is cut in half.

- *Cook your own frozen dinners.* Frozen entrees are 15 to 30 percent more expensive than similar homemade dishes. When you cook, make large amounts and freeze the leftovers in meal-size portions.

- *Buy fresh or at least frozen.* The less processed a food is, the less expensive and more nutritious it is. For vegetables, skip canned in favor of frozen, and frozen in favor of fresh (in season). Fresh broccoli at a supermarket is about 45 cents cheaper than frozen.

- *Snack on fruit.* The typical American spends $140 a year on potato chips and candy bars. Sixty-nine cents for a little bag of potato chips works out to $6 a pound! A handful of chips costs at least twice as much as piece of fruit.

Remember, the body does need some fat, although only a small amount. So, it's not a good idea to totally eliminate fat from the diet. Fat is needed for proper functioning of the body. Eliminating it altogether may do more harm than good.

Making Diet Changes: Nice and Easy Does It

Maybe you've heard the story about the woman who was upset to learn her bookstore was out of the latest "quick-weight-loss" best seller. When told it would be two weeks before the book would be available again, she was horrified. "But my class reunion is in three weeks," she moaned.

Many of us are gullible when it comes to weight loss. We know, but probably just don't want to believe, that weight loss should be the result of changing bad habits and bad diets into good habits and good diets. The changes should be permanent, not temporary fixes.

We are also prone to following some quick weight-loss program diligently for several weeks, losing the excess pounds, then reverting to our old habits. When the weight returns, we persecute ourselves, feeling guilty and losing self-esteem.

We can lose some weight on those quick-loss programs, but not fat-weight. Fat-weight doesn't come off quickly. Generally, when weight is lost quickly, that loss is water, not fat. But we shouldn't blame ourselves for failing, we should blame the quick-loss diet. It was not a good weight-loss program in the first place.

With histories of more than 40 years of creating habits behind us, it's not going to be easy to make the changes needed for permanent weight control, but it is possible. You begin by making small, easy changes over time.

Initially, it helps to keep a diet diary for several days to help identify specific problem areas. Most of us underestimate what we eat so it's very important to be exact. A sample diary is outlined below.

Dear Diary. . .

Time	Food Eaten/ Amount	Where Eaten	Activity	Mood
7 am	Bagel/1	desk	reading paper	hungry
7 am	Juice/1/2 c	desk	reading paper	hungry
11:30 am	Hamburger on bun/3 oz.	restaurant	visiting	hungry
11:30 am	French fries/20	restaurant	visiting	hungry
5:30 pm	Frozen dinner (baked chicken, green beans, apple cobbler, roll) 1	dining room	reading mail	hungry
8:30 pm	Potato chips/bag	couch	watching tv	bored

How many?

Breads/Starches	5	Vegetables	2
Meat	5 oz.	Fruits	1
Milk/Dairy	0	Extras	3

Keep Your Own Diet Diary

Day:

Time	Food Eaten/ Amount	Where Eaten	Activity	Mood
am				
pm				

How many?

Breads/Starches _____   Vegetables _____

Meat _____   Fruits _____

Milk/Dairy _____   Extras _____

Keep Your Own Diet Diary

Day:

Time	Food Eaten/ Amount	Where Eaten	Activity	Mood
am				
pm				

How many?

Breads/Starches _____   Vegetables _____

Meat _____   Fruits _____

Milk/Dairy _____   Extras _____

When using this diary, note where you tend to eat most often. Pay attention to what you are doing while you eat and how you feel. Are you eating foods from the groups on the Food Pyramid? Make it your personal challenge to fill in your own foodstyle pyramid. Identify your problem areas. Are you stomach hungry? Or are you really just mouth hungry? Are you eating out of boredom or loneliness? Are you anxious?

How about portion sizes? Do your protein portions look more like a paperback book than a deck of cards? How often do you eat? And, do you always read or watch TV when you eat?

Once you see what you are doing, you can select small steps and begin to make the changes that will secure your healthy future. If you are eating out of boredom, think about getting a new hobby. If your portions are too large, try making plates with smaller portions or use smaller salad plates instead of serving your food family style on dinner plates. Instead of reading or watching television, invite someone over to share your meal, or just enjoy the meal alone. Put your utensils down between each bite. Drink water at the table. Prepare a place setting that has visual appeal and then sit at the table and savor it.

Choose romaine lettuce over iceberg. One cup provides about 20% of the daily requirement of beta carotene and twice the fiber as iceberg lettuce.

Attack each behavior you want to change individually. Start with a goal of one behavior a week. Maybe that means eliminating your evening snack. Or perhaps it's using fruit spread on your bagel instead of butter, or drinking low-fat milk instead of whole milk.

Once you are accustomed to that change, make another change. Incorporate a brisk walk into your day, even if it means parking further from your office or the grocery store. Remember each and every change brings you a step closer to that healthy lifestyle that will enable you to enjoy the years to come.

Out with the Old, In with the New

Here's our list of the best tips for changing bad eating habits:

- Plan your meals and snacks in advance. Know what you are planning to eat before you raid the refrigerator or pantry in a panic.

- Shop for groceries after you've eaten, not before. You won't be tempted to buy things you don't really want if you are full. Also, prepare a grocery list and stick to it.

- Assign specific eating areas in your home and only eat there. The kitchen and dining room are the usual choices. Always sit down when you are eating.

- Make eating a singular activity. Don't combine eating with reading or television watching. Pay attention to what you are eating.

- Serve meals on smaller plates. This technique makes it look like you have a lot more food than you really have and works well when combined with the technique of setting your utensils down between bites.

- Take your time while you eat. Because it takes 20 minutes for your stomach to signal your brain that you are full, enjoy eating slowly. Don't rush through your meals, then feel overstuffed later. It is a fact that thin people eat more slowly than heavy people.

- Dish plates up at the stove, rather than serving the meal family style and putting full serving dishes on the table. You are less likely to want seconds this way. Remember, when you opt for second helpings, you are really eating another entire meal—that's two at one seating.

- Get out of the kitchen. Find other places to "hang out." Use the kitchen for meal preparation and eating, not for chatting on the telephone or socializing with friends and family.

- Choose foods that take longer to eat. Fresh fruits and vegetables take longer to eat and you can actually enjoy them more than, for example, drinking a glass of juice.

- Be sensible when you eat out. Choose restaurants that can provide you with the types of food you want. Avoid "All-You-Can-Eat" buffets. They are simply too tempting.

- Stay in control of social situations. Don't lean on the appetizer table. Move around, mingle, and enjoy the company.

- Don't eat when you are feeling stressed. Take a walk or a bath instead.

- Don't be obsessed with the bathroom scale. All you need for good control is to step on the scale once a week. Choose the same day each week, and the same time of day.

Realistically, a weight loss of 1 to 2 pounds a week is a safe goal. To lose 1 pound, you have to burn off 3,500 calories. In an average person, a deficit of 500 calories per day usually results in the loss of 1 pound of fat per week, accomplished either by eating fewer calories or burning more calories by exercising, or by combining both. Of course, if you take in 3,500 more calories than you use up, the net effect will be adding a pound of fat. There is a wide variable in the amounts of calories people can eat to maintain certain body weights.

Some women do lose more than 1 to 2 pounds per week, especially when they first begin a weight-reduction program. This is not uncommon since the body is adjusting to the dietary change. Of course, water can account for some of this loss. Eventually, the weight loss will slow down, but it will continue if an adequate weight-reduction plan is followed.

Physical activity, as we said, can accelerate weight loss since it burns calories. A combination, therefore, of reducing your food intake and increasing your exercise sets the stage for the best results at the losing game.

Losing weight can be difficult, however, and it should never be treated as a short-term solution to a lifetime problem. Your ultimate goal should be to establish healthful habits, to learn more about nutrition, and to eliminate any self-defeating behaviors that can impede your progress.

Here's our list of tips for challenging and changing those old habits. Practicing these new behaviors can lead you into a new, healthy food-style all your own.

Make Your Goal Health, Not Dieting

Many women look for the quick fix. Eating healthy sounds a lot easier than it really is; we recognize that. Use the Food Pyramid as your guide. Select the right number of servings from each group. When making your choices, think about the following:

- Choose low-calorie, low-fat, nutritious foods in moderate amounts from each group on the food pyramid.

- Remember the key words: variety and moderation. Opt for more complex carbohydrates, dried beans and peas, fresh fruits and vegetables, low-fat dairy products, and lean meats. Here's a reminder list of foods from which to choose.

Choosy Eaters Pick . . .

Group	Best Choices	Choose these Less Often
Meat, Protein	lean meat, poultry, fish, egg whites, dried beans, peas, legumes	fatty meats, organ meat, processed and luncheon meats, egg yolks, chicken skin
Milk, Dairy	low-fat or nonfat milk, cottage cheese, yogurt, frozen yogurt, cheese	whole milk or milk products made with whole milk, ice cream

Choosy Eaters Pick, continued

Group	Best Choices	Choose these Less Often
Fruits, Vegetables	fresh, frozen, canned, or dried	any fruit or vegetable prepared in or covered in sauce, butter, or cream
Breads, Cereals	whole wheat, whole grain breads and cereals, crackers, pasta, rice, couscous	croissants, buttered rolls, pastries, snack crackers, granola cereals, pasta or rice made with butter or cream sauces
Fats, Oils	unsaturated vegetable oil like Canola, olive, sunflower, peanut, safflower, soybean, or sesame; low-fat salad dressing and mayo	butter, coconut oil, palm oil, high-fat salad dressing and mayo
Snacks	sherbet, low-fat frozen yogurt, popsicles, low-fat or nonfat cookies, cakes, popcorn, pretzels	ice cream, candy, chocolate, pie, frosted cakes, fried chips

- Make every bite count. Eat slowly and enjoy.
- Start with your Diet Diary today. Remember, tomorrow never really ever comes. Every day is a challenge, but keep going. Stick with it! You can conquer this and you'll be glad you did.

- Avoid fad diets. Although it's tempting to all of us, avoid fad diets. Don't aim for short-term solutions. They will cost you more in the end, both in money and in health.

- Move more. Exercise and physical activity helps burn excess calories, increase metabolism, control appetite, and makes you feel really good about yourself.

Sample Menu Plan

See how your changes can work in a 1200 calorie, low-fat menu plan. Here's a two-day sample plan for you to use as a model.

Day 1	Serving Size	Calories	Fat (gm)
Breakfast			
chilled orange juice	1/2 cup	54	0
hard-cooked egg	1	77	5
whole wheat bagel	1/2	71	0
margarine	1 tsp.	34	4
2% milk	1 cup	121	5
Lunch			
sandwich of—			
sliced turkey	2 oz.	79	1
on whole wheat bread	2 slices	172	3
fat-free mayonnaise	1 Tbsp.	11	0
lettuce leaves	2	5	0
tomato slices	2	6	0
fresh apple	81	0	0

Sample Menu Plan Day 1, continued

	Serving Size	Calories	Fat (gm)
Dinner			
poached swordfish	4 oz.	174	6
with lemon juice	1 tsp.	1	0
baked sweet potato	1	117	0
steamed fresh broccoli	2 spears	21	0
tossed green salad	1 cup	25	0
with French dressing	1 Tbsp.	70	6
low-calorie cherry gelatin cubes	1/2 cup	0	0
Snack			
banana milkshake made with—			
banana	1/2	52	0
2% milk	1 cup	121	5
Total		***1211 calories***	***35 gm fat***

Sample Menu Plan

Day 2	Serving Size	Calories	Fat (gm)
Breakfast			
hot cooked oatmeal	1/2 cup	72	1
with raisins	1 Tbsp.	27	0
2% milk	1 cup	121	5
Lunch			
chicken Caesar salad made with—			
romaine lettuce	1 cup	9	0
cooked, sliced breast of chicken	3/4 cup	106	2
Parmesan cheese	1 Tbsp.	28	2
Caesar salad dressing	1 Tbsp.	52	5
hard white roll	1	147	2
margarine	1 tsp.	34	4
Dinner			
hamburger	3 oz.	275	12
on bun	1	129	2
with lettuce leaves	2	5	0
and tomato	2 slices	6	0
dill pickle	1	12	0
fresh steamed green beans	1/2 cup	22	0
fresh carrot/celery sticks	1 each	37	0
chilled cantaloupe melon	1/8 melon	23	0

Sample Menu Plan Day 2, *continued*

	Serving Size	Calories	Fat (gm)
Snack			
graham cracker	1	30	1
2% milk	1 cup	121	5
Total		**1256 calories**	**41 gm fat**

Foods to Stay Vibrant, Young & Healthy

4

Exercise:

A Key to Better Health

If you saw a product advising, "Follow instructions properly and lose weight, live longer, feel better, reduce stress, sleep better, have firmer thighs and a flatter tummy, tone muscle, and reduce your risk of diabetes, cardiovascular disease, and high blood pressure," you'd want to rush out and get it, right? Well, as you can probably guess by this chapter's subject, it's not a product at all. It's exercise. And it costs nothing at all.

If it's really that good, why doesn't everybody take advantage of exercise and reap its benefits. Well, too many of us just don't. And, we think up excuses to avoid it. Did you realize that more than 60 percent of the adult American population does not get enough exercise?

Many women remain sedentary, thinking that exercise has to be difficult and unpleasant to do us any good. Overall fitness can become your goal later, but for right now, just take a walk. It's definitely worth your while. Any exercise is better than none.

In this chapter, we want to show you how to get moving, if you aren't already. And if you are, we'll help you improve on your current exercise program.

> *Buy tuna packed in water instead of oil and you'll reduce the fat from 7 grams to less than 1 per 3-ounce serving. That's half a 6 1/2-ounce can.*
>
> ~

But why a discussion on exercise in a book about food and nutrition, you may ask. In a nutshell, a good foodstyle will go a long way in promoting a healthy life, but it is not until you combine it with exercise that you can achieve true vibrancy. By the same token, even a vigorous exercise program will be for naught if you do not have a healthy foodstyle; the two work best together.

A Beneficial Union

As we age, we tend to tire more easily. We seem to have less energy to even think about becoming more active. But once we understand the health benefits and realize that we can feel better and live longer by programming some exercise into our lives, exercise becomes very attractive.

The three most common questions women ask about exercise are:

1. What kind of exercise should I be doing?
2. How often should I exercise?
3. How can I stay motivated to keep it up?

Exercise improves your overall health, and:

- you can begin an exercise program no matter what age you start and you'll still benefit from it.
- daily exercise throughout life adds to the quality of that life.
- active individuals tend to be nonsmokers and to eat more healthfully.
- regular exercise helps reduce your risk of cancer, diabetes, cardiovascular disease, high blood pressure, obesity, and depression.
- exercise helps lower your cholesterol level and improves your muscle tone and flexibility.
- exercise helps reduce side effects of premenstrual syndrome (PMS) and menopause.

Exercise fights fat, and:

- walking longer than 20 minutes at a time allows fat to be burned more rapidly.
- increasing your exercise, in combination with limiting your fat and calorie intake, acts as the best method for reducing overall body weight.
- regular aerobic exercise (exercise that increases your heart rate over a period of time) increases your body metabolism, not only during exercise, but afterwards as well. This increases the calories your body burns all day long.

Exercise benefits you psychologically and emotionally by:

- helping you to deal with stress.
- increasing your self-confidence and self-esteem and making you feel and look better.
- taking you away from the stresses of the world, even if only for a little while.

What Kind of Exercise is Best?

The greatest health benefits result from a combination of aerobic exercise, resistance training, and stretching, so these three elements should be part of your personal fitness program. But increasing your physical activity anyway you can is a start.

Aerobic exercise increases your heart rate over time. Many people confuse aerobic exercise with aerobic dancing and don't even get started. Although aerobic dancing is a type of aerobic exercise, it's not the only option. It is very important to find an exercise that you enjoy. If you like it, you'll stick with it. If one type is not for you, look for another.

Use a vegetable oil or olive-oil flavored cooking spray to coat cooking and baking utensils. You'll be using 90 percent fewer calories than if you used butter, margarine, or oil.

Aerobic exercises use large muscles and provide for continuous rhythmic movements that help raise your heart level. These exercises usually involve the entire body, condition the heart and lungs, reduce risks for diabetes and obesity, and increase the oxygen supply to all parts of the body.

With aerobic exercise, you'll work hard enough to raise your heart rate. You'll break a sweat, but you won't feel winded or out of breath. After you get in shape, you'll feel relaxed and energized following exercise. Some examples of aerobic exercise include walking, jogging, stair climbing, dancing, biking, and jumping rope.

Aerobic exercise should be the key element in your exercise program. But, make sure to include a 10-minute warmup with stretching and calisthenics and a 5-minute cool down of walking and stretching after the aerobic exercise.

Jogging and running are more intense than walking, which is a plus since you get a better workout in less time. The negative side, especially for midlife women, is that the bones and joints of the body are subjected to substantial impact. If you don't enjoy jogging or running, you aren't likely to stick with either.

> *Have questions about fitness?*
>
> *The Aerobics and Fitness Foundation answers questions regarding safe and effective exercise programs and practices. Call (800) 233-4486.*

Swimming and water aerobics are the least traumatic for the body. That is, they have the least impact on our joints as water absorbs 90 percent of the force of gravity, providing cushioning and protection. Swimming involves the entire body and improves flexibility. It is the best exercise for arthritis sufferers. It does not, however, help you to build or retain bone, something of vital importance to midlife women.

Biking can vary in intensity, from gentle exercise to marathon racing. Bikers need to bike at least three times the distance as a walker or runner goes to achieve the same aerobic benefit.

Aerobic dancing uses all muscle groups and motivates you with music. You also are likely to stay interested by learning new routines and by interacting with other members of the group. A fixed class schedule is good for some women and too rigid for others, so find the right program if this sounds like the one for you. Some women prefer the scheduling flexibility offered by exercise shows on television or videotapes.

Resistance training, which uses weights and elastic bands, provides muscle strength, tones specific muscle groups, and increases muscle endurance. We become stronger using resistance training by applying force against a resistance. These exercises aren't as good as aerobic exercises in burning fat, but they are good for improving body shape and tone and for fighting osteoporosis.

Preventing loss of strength becomes very important as we age. Although we can't yet stop the aging process, we can slow it down by staying fit. Much of the decrease in physical strength observed in many older women is a direct result of a sedentary lifestyle. Women who sit become weak and lose their ability to carry out the essential tasks such as grocery shopping, meal preparation, and light housekeeping that enable them to remain independent. Some researchers believe that regular exercise and resistance training can postpone age-related loss of function by 10 to 20 years. We can truly say exercise is the "fountain of youth."

Stretching promotes adequate joint flexibility, which, in turn, prevents injury and chronic muscular or skeletal problems that result in low-back pain, among other discomforts. Like strength, flexibility can decline with age, so regular stretching should be used to slow down that stiffness that creeps up on us with age.

Stretching is easy to learn, but there is a right and wrong way to stretch. Your doctor should be able to recommend an exercise specialist or book to teach proper stretching and exercise techniques. In general, though, the right way is a sustained, relaxed stretch in which you feel mild tension. Each stretch should be held for 10 to 30 seconds at a time. Breathing should be slow, controlled, and rhythmic. Don't hold your

> *Antioxidants (vitamins E and selenium) in wheat germ and other foods are thought to protect against various forms of cancer. In addition, high-fiber wheat germ helps regulate bowel function and offers protection against colon and rectal cancers.*

breath while you stretch. The more you stretch, the more flexible you will become. Bouncing while you stretch or stretching until you hurt should be avoided.

How Often Should I Exercise?

The benefits of exercise do not last forever. In fact, runners often lose their training effect in a few weeks. So you must continue exercising to keep on reaping the benefits over the long haul. Exercising every other day, or four times a week, is considered the minimum for any exercise benefits at all. Thirty minutes a day of moderate activity is another approach.

Many women think they just don't have time for this, but review how much time you really have for less active pursuits. How much time do you spend on the telephone? How about watching television? Try to put your body to work as much as possible—every little bit will help. Be persistent, but not impatient. You are building a program to last your lifetime—that's a marathon, not a 50-yard dash!

How Much is Enough?

Health and fitness experts recommend the following schedule as the minimum. This is the "ideal," but, remember, the best fitness program is the one that works for you and the one you will continue.

Aerobic exercise	*3 to 5 times per week* 20 to 60 minutes per session at medium effort (50 to 70 percent maximum heart rate)
Resistance training	*2 times per week* 8 to 12 repetitions of 8 to 10 different exercises each, covering all the major muscle groups
Stretching	*3 to 5 times per week*

As you become adjusted to a specific exercise program, you may want to increase the length of time and the intensity of your exercise. Keep challenging your body . . . that's one road to lifetime fitness.

Motor Up Your Motivation

It's always difficult to get motivated to do something you know you should do but you don't really want to do. First, you really do have to want it. Once you commit yourself to beginning an exercise program, you will need to set some small goals. Overdoing it right at the start will cause pain, pain will discourage you, and your commitment won't last.

Let's say you choose to begin with a walking program. Commit to yourself that you'll walk around the block three days the first week. In the second or third week, go twice around the block when you walk. If you start small and add more as time goes on, your goals will be achievable and you'll succeed. Nothing helps you feel better about yourself than success at achieving your own goals.

To reduce fat in casseroles, use sharp cheddar on the top for flavor and fill the middle with mozzarella or another low-fat cheese.

After a while, walking becomes great fun; you'll begin to enjoy it and look forward to it. You could also find a friend to join you. Many women find it easier to work out if they are doing it with a buddy. If you're committed, you'll both look forward to walking, talking, and sharing progress together. And, when one drags her feet, the other can offer encouragement. Once you begin to see results, you'll simply want to continue, so motivation becomes another benefit of your program.

Remember, it all begins with a single step. Start slowly. Aim for slow, steady progress. As Shakespeare said, "Too swift arrives as tardy as too slow!"

Start Slowly to Live Strong

- If you have any questions about your health, check with your doctor before you start your exercise program. For women over 40, we recommend an exercise stress test. Don't start a rigorous exercise program if you haven't had a medical checkup in the last year.

- Walking is a great way to start to increase your activity level. Start with some easy stretching, then some walking, followed by a cool down period. Your cool down should be some slower walking. End your session with more stretches. You may not even break a sweat in the first week, but starting slowly helps give your body a chance to adjust to the new routine, and you'll avoid having sore muscles. After two or three days, you may want to take a day off to give your body time to adjust.

- Your rate of exercise depends on your current physical condition. If you are inactive, a walk around the block or just up to the corner may be a workout in itself. If you are in good physical condition, exercising may be a bit more easy.

- Exercise at your own pace. Walk one block or cycle one mile instead of trying to go miles the first day. You'll be more apt to develop good exercise habits if you set small realizable goals in the beginning. Also, risk of injury is less if you start slowly and move at your own pace.

- Listen to your body. Signs of over-exertion include pounding in your chest, shortness of breath, dizziness, excessive sweating, and faintness. Slow down and cool off for 5 to 10 minutes at the end of your exercise. If symptoms persist, see your doctor.

- Use the "talk test" to judge whether you're exercising too hard. If you can't talk while you exercise, you're overdoing it.

- Choose an exercise you enjoy. Any heart-raising activity is good. Easy strolling, very brisk walking, stepping, aerobic dance, swimming, water aerobics, rope jumping, biking, or rowing are all good exercises.

- Choose exercises that are best for you. Consider your body build, your finances, your overall health, and your athletic experience.
- Exercise safely. Walk or jog facing traffic or on a walking trail. Bike with traffic, but avoid busy roads. Wear a helmet. Go with a friend.

As we've said, walking is a wonderful aerobic exercise. It's appropriate for people of all ages, safe, and does not cost a thing. If you want to begin a walking program, as with any other program, start slowly. Your goal is not only to exercise, but to enjoy yourself. Here's how you can get started.

Week	Warm Up	Brisk Walking	Cool Down	Total
1	5 minutes	5 minutes	5 minutes	15
2	5 minutes	7 minutes	5 minutes	17
3	5 minutes	9 minutes	5 minutes	19
4	5 minutes	11 minutes	5 minutes	21
5	5 minutes	13 minutes	5 minutes	23
6	5 minutes	15 minutes	5 minutes	25
7	5 minutes	18 minutes	5 minutes	28
8	5 minutes	20 minutes	5 minutes	30
9	5 minutes	23 minutes	5 minutes	33
10	5 minutes	26 minutes	5 minutes	36
11	5 minutes	28 minutes	5 minutes	38
12	5 minutes	30 minutes	5 minutes	40

Time is On Your Side

As we said, many women just don't think they have time for exercise. Exercise may take a one-hour chunk out of your day and so it probably requires some planning to schedule time for it into your hectic lifestyle.

Finding ways to incorporate exercise into your current activity is an alternative to carving out a specific hour in the day for your fitness program. Sometimes, four 15-minute sessions a day may be just as beneficial.

- Early morning may be the best time for women with young families who have little free time. Try waking up an hour earlier (or even a half hour) and then working out with an exercise video or television exercise show.

- Get in the habit of exercising at a certain time of the day. Having a special time to exercise helps you stay away from distractions like television, housework, shopping, or the like. Take care of yourself before you take care of other things.

- Break the monotony. If you walk, map out several routes in your neighborhood, on a walking path, or in the mall. Determine each distance and how long it takes you to get from your starting point to the end. Having several routes makes it more interesting and increases your chances of sticking with it. Take a friend along for moral support. Interesting conversation makes the time pass quickly. If a friend is not available, how about listening to music or a book-on-tape on your "walkman." Just make sure you can still hear any approaching cars and other potential hazards.

- Set your priorities. Exercise and fitness are basic to your health. Schedule time for exercise as if you are making an appointment or play date for yourself or your child. It's certainly as important! Health is our most precious possession, even if we never realize it until it is lost. Ask yourself when you have a cold or the flu what you would do to feel good again. Chances are getting some exercise now will help you stave off even colds and flu.

To lighten up recipes, use dairy products with reduced fat content such as low-fat or skim milk, low-fat or nonfat yogurt, and light sour cream. Use evaporated skim milk instead of heavy cream in quiches, creamy soups, and other dishes that call for milk or cream.

- Include fitness into your everyday routine. Move more during your day wherever you are. Take the stairs instead of riding elevators or escalators. Park in the back of the parking lot instead of right up front. Move around your house or office while you talk on the phone. Walk to a farther bus stop or get off earlier and walk the distance. Take daily walks during your lunch breaks. Or take your child for a walk or a ride on the back of your bicycle. Baby joggers can be a good investment if you are expanding your family.

- Make social fitness dates. Instead of making social plans that include lunch, happy hour, dinner, or a movie, plan tennis or racquetball games, biking or hiking dates, or just walks in the park. You'll feel better and enjoy your company just the same.

- If you have the opportunity to join a health club, take advantage of various types of equipment. Have an exercise physiologist or trainer demonstrate equipment first and set up a specific plan for you.

- Choose several different forms of exercise. Switch from walking to cycling to mall walking to swimming to water aerobics just to keep from getting bored and to avoid possible injury. Exercising different muscles with different activities is better for your body than using the same muscles and joints over and over.

- Dress comfortably. Loose fitting or light clothes in warm and humid climates permit heat loss; hats, gloves, and warm clothes help keep the heat in on cold days in cold places. Wear a proper support or sports bra, if needed. You don't have to look like a fashion model when you walk.

- Carry a water bottle. Drink plenty of water before, during, and after exercise, particularly in warm weather.

- Adjust your schedule to the weather. Don't push yourself in heat and humidity, and don't venture out in extremely cold or rainy weather.

Remember, you have to get up to shape up. What have you got to lose but fat, stress, sagging muscles, and other health problems? You'll become fitter, happier, healthier, and more productive when you become a regular exerciser.

Baby Your Feet

Are you amazed how many types of athletic shoes there are? Can you even begin to look for the best ones to suit your needs and lifestyle? Here's our list of tips:

- Look for good cushioning when planning to buy shoes for jogging or running. Remember those exercises require shock absorption.

- Walking shoes are not appropriate for running, but running shoes can be worn for walking.

- Heel cushions and flexible soles are important in a walking shoe.

- Aerobic dance shoes should have good support and cushioned with flexible soles.

- Specific sports require specific shoes (baseball, football, bowling, golf, and the like). Seek assistance when you need it.

- Buy name brands.

- Make sure the shoes feel good, fit right, and provide the comfort you need to enjoy your sport. Seek attention for blisters or sores that don't heal.

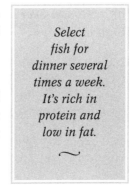

Select fish for dinner several times a week. It's rich in protein and low in fat.

Exercise Intensity

As you begin to work out on a regular basis, you'll notice that the intensity of your exercise increases. This is obvious to you when you note changes in your breathing, how much you sweat, and how tired you feel. It's important to increase the intensity of your exercise, but it is also smart to understand what your limits are.

You should be aware of your heart rate during your workout. Individual heart monitors are available but expensive. The talking test, mentioned earlier (can you talk without sounding winded?), is another good check. Or, you can use the chart that follows on the "Rate of Perceived Exertion."

To determine how you rate, locate your pulse on the thumb side of your wrist. Take your pulse for 6 seconds and multiply that number by 10 to get your actual heart rate. If that number is far above your target heart rate, slow down. If it is far below, speed up. Checking your heart rate should be a routine part of aerobic activity. Calculate your target heart rate by using the formula below.

Estimating Target Heart Rate

220 - _____ = _____
     (your age)   (maximum heart rate)

For a woman over age 50 who is just beginning a physical fitness program

_____ x .50 (or 50%) = _____
(max. heart rate)   (target heart rate)

For a woman over age 40 just beginning a physical fitness program

_____ x .60 (or 60%) = _____
(max. heart rate)   (target heart rate)

For a woman over 40 who is in fair to good condition

_____ x .75 (or 75%) = _____
(max. heart rate)   (target heart rate)

Any woman who is in excellent condition

_____ x .80 (or 80%) = _____
(max. heart rate)   (target heart rate)

Rate of Perceived Exertion

The following scale rates the intensity of your workout by assigning a number from 0 to 10 to represent how you are feeling during the exercise. Numbers 3 to 6 are in the healthy range.

Number	Definition of Number	Target Zone
0	Nothing at all	
0.5	Very, very weak	
1	Very weak	
2	Weak	
3	Moderate *(feel comfortable but can continue for long period)*	60% of maximum heart rate
4	Somewhat strong *(a little heavy breathing)*	70% of maximum heart rate
5	Strong *(breathing accelerated, hard)*	80% of maximum heart rate
6	Strong *(fast breathing—feel like you can continue, very hard)*	85% of maximum heart rate
7	Very strong *(heavy breathing)*	

Number	Definition of Number	Target Zone
8	Breathless	
9	Very breathless	
10	Very, very strong *(extreme breathlessness, extreme burning in muscles)*	maximum heart rate

Exercise vs. Dieting for Weight Loss: The Victor Is . . .

Exercise may be more effective than dieting for losing body fat. For years, dieting by drastically cutting calories has been the first option, and often the only option, for losing weight. This was especially true for women. And, more often than not, after a short time, weight loss slacks off, the dieter gets frustrated and resumes her old eating habits and the weight comes back, plus. Then, the woman dieter ends up with a higher percentage of body fat than she started with. Why does this happen?

Dieting (calorie restriction) and exercise (calorie burning) have different effects on the metabolic rate of the human body.

Severe calorie restriction (that is very low calorie diets of 800 calories or less) over long periods decreases the body's basal metabolic rate. That is the number of calories needed just to sustain the body's basic processes. Severe food restriction also causes loss of lean muscle tissue. Muscle loss can occur even on sensible diet plans, particularly when exercise is not incorporated into the program.

On the other hand, regular exercise increases the metabolic rate of the body by increasing lean muscle mass. Often, the body's metabolism may remain "revved up" for as much as 6 to 24 hours after a 30-minute exercise session. This increase in calories burned is often called the "afterglow" of exercise and could, by itself, result in a weight loss of 4 to 5 pounds in a year (based on 30 minutes of exercise done 5 to 6 times per week).

Exercise may also be a mild appetite suppressant, primarily for those who participate in light to moderate exercise for up to one hour daily. Many sedentary women often eat slightly more than women who exercise regularly.

In order to lose body fat (not muscle), a calorie deficit of 100 to 500 calories per day is needed.

> *To cut calories in half, use fresh fruit, juice-packed canned fruit, or frozen unsweetened fruit instead of canned fruit in heavy syrup.*

By increasing exercise or by exercising longer, more intensely, or more days per week, dieters can eat adequate calories and still achieve weight (or fat) loss.

Sometimes, however, the results don't show up on the bathroom scale because with exercise there is some minor weight gain as a result of increased muscle mass. Muscle tissue weighs more than fat tissue, so perhaps a better measure of your success, at least during the starting weeks of your program, is the looser fit of your clothes. Shaping up is another good way to show the positive changes that are taking place in your body.

Making Workouts Homework

Thanks to technology, exercise equipment has advanced from barbells to high-tech machinery. Some home-gym equipment even resembles the workout you get at a full-service health club. Whether you prefer sweating it out in your own home or the camaraderie at the health club, gym equipment can help you achieve your fitness goals.

But what kind of equipment is good and what is not? Which machines work and which don't? Here's our advice: Before you buy any equipment,

> *Don't chop too much. The more you chop vegetables, the more vitamins and minerals they lose. Also, try not to discard dark green outer leaves or stems. It's here where most of the vitamins and minerals are concentrated.*
>
> ~

try out a variety to determine which you like the most. Any reputable store will work with you to test equipment prior to purchase. Beware of mail order products, however, that look tempting on television or in magazines.

We have evaluated various home fitness devices for you below. As with any major purchase, however, research the item thoroughly before you invest. Home exercise equipment can often be compared to the typical female body—underused! Annually Americans invest more than $2 billion in exercise machines. All machines offer great benefits, but only if used regularly—and we don't mean used for hanging laundry on!

Using home equipment can help you save time, too. You can watch the TV news, read a newspaper or book, or talk with a friend or colleague while you pedal your home cycle or step the time away.

The following information categorizes many types of home equipment. All are convenient; most take little skill, produce few injuries, and have ranges from beginner to elite athlete. See what might work best for you.

The Ins and Outs of Exercise Equipment

Treadmills—
Walking briskly or on a slight incline on a treadmill is one of the best overall indoor activities. The easy-to-use, low impact machines provide good aerobic benefits. Treadmills range from $500 to $4000, although inexpensive models may be noisy and easily breakable. Electronic models should be easy to control and have an accessible on/off switch. The

walking belt should also be wide enough to walk comfortably. Before purchasing, be sure to measure the machine and space available at home. Allow an extra 1 foot on sides, 2 feet in back, and space for head room. Choose speed range of 1 to 6 mph for walking and 1 to 12 mph for jogging.

Stair Climbers—

This low impact machine not only improves aerobic capacity, it strengthens and firms hips, thighs, buttocks, and legs. On top of this, it is a great calorie burner. Models range from $200 to $3500, with special features such as feedback on number of steps, steps per minute, calories used, and preset programs. Just make sure the model you choose has a stable, sturdy frame and the features you want. Also, before purchasing, measure the space it will require, allowing extra space for head room. A stair climber is easy to use, but be sure to start at low intensity.

Cross Country Ski Machines—

One of the best forms of aerobic exercise that uses both arms and legs, these machines provide no-impact activity. Machines cost between $100 to $1500 on average and come in various sizes. Many are collapsible for easy storage, although all require coordination and practice to move one foot forward while the opposite arm moves back. Practice before you purchase and choose a machine with smooth motion and one that you can coordinate.

Stationary Bicycles—

These low impact, easy-to-use machines provide aerobic benefits and primarily work the lower body. Some models, however, include a "dual action" upper body arm workout plus muscle toning. A semi-reclining recumbent bike will support the low back and keep blood pressure lower. Stationary bicycles range in price from $200 to $3500 and come in many sizes. Newer models track time, distance, speed, calories used, and heart rate, and offer variable resistance levels. Whichever model you choose, make sure it feels good to you, is comfortable, and easy to peddle. A well padded and adjustable seat is a must.

Rowing Machines—

Offering a low impact aerobic activity, rowing machines are great for toning muscles in the arms and upper body. Styles are based on air or water resistance and cost between $300 and $3500. Many are 8-feet long. Choose one that feels good to you and concentrate on making your strokes smooth.

Multi-Gyms and Multi-Station Weight Training Machines—

These machines offer a variety of setups to lift weights and exercise the entire body. Benefits include muscle toning and improved strength, endurance, and flexibility. They offer the safest way to lift weights without a spotter and can also protect the lower back better than free weights. Machines range from $300 to $5000 and require ample space. Look for models with smooth cables and fluent lifting action. Begin at low weights and increase gradually.

Free Weights—

Dumbbells and other free weights help tone muscles and build strength. Costing $0.40 to $0.60 per pound, free weights are easy to use, but you should get some instruction for safe methods. Begin at low weights.

Heart Rate Monitors—

These wrist watch-type monitors are worn directly on the body and provide continuous heart rate readings. This information helps in tracking total exercise spent in your target heart zone. Models average between $200 and $300.

Exercise Videos—

There are a large variety of exercise videos, ranging from low to high impact aerobics and others that emphasize muscle strengthening or flexibility. They cost between $10 and $50.

Plan Your Exercise

To help you get started with scheduling exercise into your life, we present a 12-week planner on the following pages. Start off by planning what you will do. Congratulate yourself when you do it. Then you'll find yourself filling in the chart after the fact. Once that happens, you'll know you're on your way to gathering all the benefits that exercise provides.

Week 1

Monday	Tuesday	Wednesday	Thursday	Friday	Sat/Sun
Time:	Time:	Time:	Time:	Time:	Time:
Activity	Activity	Activity	Activity	Activity	Activity

Week 2

Monday	Tuesday	Wednesday	Thursday	Friday	Sat/Sun
Time:	Time:	Time:	Time:	Time:	Time:
Activity	Activity	Activity	Activity	Activity	Activity

Week 3

Monday	Tuesday	Wednesday	Thursday	Friday	Sat/Sun
Time:	Time:	Time:	Time:	Time:	Time:
Activity	Activity	Activity	Activity	Activity	Activity

Week 4

Time:	Time:	Time:	Time:	Time:	Time:
Activity	Activity	Activity	Activity	Activity	Activity

Week 5

Monday	Tuesday	Wednesday	Thursday	Friday	Sat/Sun
Time: Activity	Time: Activity	Time: Activity	Time: Activity	Time: Activity	Time: Activity

Week 6

Monday	Tuesday	Wednesday	Thursday	Friday	Sat/Sun
Time: Activity	Time: Activity	Time: Activity	Time: Activity	Time: Activity	Time: Activity

Foods to Stay Vibrant, Young & Healthy

Week 7

Monday	Tuesday	Wednesday	Thursday	Friday	Sat/Sun
Time:	Time:	Time:	Time:	Time:	Time:
Activity	Activity	Activity	Activity	Activity	Activity

Week 8

Monday	Tuesday	Wednesday	Thursday	Friday	Sat/Sun
Time:	Time:	Time:	Time:	Time:	Time:
Activity	Activity	Activity	Activity	Activity	Activity

Week 9

Monday	Tuesday	Wednesday	Thursday	Friday	Sat/Sun
Time:	Time:	Time:	Time:	Time:	Time:
Activity	Activity	Activity	Activity	Activity	Activity

Week 10

Monday	Tuesday	Wednesday	Thursday	Friday	Sat/Sun
Time:	Time:	Time:	Time:	Time:	Time:
Activity	Activity	Activity	Activity	Activity	Activity

Week 11

Monday	Tuesday	Wednesday	Thursday	Friday	Sat/Sun
Time:	Time:	Time:	Time:	Time:	Time:
Activity	Activity	Activity	Activity	Activity	Activity

Week 12

Monday	Tuesday	Wednesday	Thursday	Friday	Sat/Sun
Time:	Time:	Time:	Time:	Time:	Time:
Activity	Activity	Activity	Activity	Activity	Activity

Foods to Stay Vibrant, Young & Healthy

5

Getting Organized:

Planning Meals
and Menus

A re you organized in every area of your life but the kitchen? Do you keep a "Daytimer" pocket calendar or organizer, know every birthday, business meeting, and date of your grandson's soccer games? Yet you get home at 5:00 pm and don't have the energy to plan, let alone cook, dinner.

Okay, you probably pop a frozen dinner in the microwave. Or maybe you phone the local Chinese restaurant or pizza palace and have dinner delivered. Possibly you just let everyone fend for themselves and you raid the cupboard for anything that's there. If this describes you, it's time to get your foodstyle as organized as the rest of your life.

Weight-conscious women tend to love weight-loss programs that plan everything out for them. In fact, the companies that supply the food as well as the plan have a real gold mine going for them. But for most of us, the day comes when we need to take back the reins.

> *When making 2 or 3-egg omeletes, substitute 2 egg whites for a single whole egg. You'll save 55 calories and eliminate at least 200 milligrams of cholesterol. You can also substitute 2 egg whites for a whole egg in baking.*

Planning meals isn't a high priority for many busy midlife women. Most of us are lucky to grab a cup of coffee and muffin as we dash out the door in the morning. How do you put "balance" into that kind of lifestyle?

Well, let's think back to the Food Guide Pyramid. If you are a woman whose hectic lifestyle dictates assistance in putting together the "right stuff" for your foodstyle, we have a plan to help you.

Serve it Tasty, Fast, and Nutritious

The recipes of the 1940s, '50s, and '60s, were heavier in fat content than today's lighter and leaner cuisine. Probably as a response to the

"Depression Years," it was also thought that bigger portions of the main course—the beef, chicken, or pork roast—and smaller servings of side dishes was the way to go. The goal, of course, was to look "fat and prosperous."

Today we know it should be just the opposite—larger portions of pasta, rice, and salad, and small servings of chicken, fish, or beef should be the goal.

In the following pages, you'll find a week's worth of menus based on the needs of less physically active women. Each day's food provides about 1600 calories and less than 30 percent of those calories are from fat.

Plan a meatless main meal at least once a week to reduce fat and increase protein, fiber, and iron. Good options include legumes, kidney beans, lima beans, garbanzo beans, lentils, and peas.

For women who may have a need for increased calories, those who are extremely physically active, look back at the recommended number of servings on the food pyramid and increase your foods, snacks, or portion sizes accordingly. If you are interested in dropping a few pounds, decrease your food choices, snacks, and portion sizes, and try to lower your fat intake even more than these samples.

7-Day Menu Sampler

Day 1	Serving Size	Calories	Fat (gm)
Breakfast			
chilled orange slices	1 orange	62	0
wheat bran muffin	1	124	4
margarine	1 tsp.	34	4
2% milk	1 cup	121	5
Lunch			
sliced breast of turkey	3 oz.	119	1
on whole wheat bread	2 slices	172	3
with mayonnaise	1 Tbsp.	11	0
lettuce leaves	2	5	0
tomato	2 slices	6	0
carrot and celery sticks	1 stick/stalk	37	0
vanilla wafers	6	106	4
Dinner			
broiled dilled salmon with lemon wedge	4 oz.	206	9
pilaf of brown rice	3/4 cup	162	1
with mushrooms	1/2 cup	19	0
margarine	1 tsp.	34	4
steamed fresh asparagus	6 spears	22	0

Day 1 (continued)	Serving Size	Calories	Fat (gm)
Dinner (continued)			
fresh spinach salad	1 cup	89	4
low-fat salad dressing	1 Tbsp.	16	1
fresh apple slices	1 medium apple	81	0
Snack			
fresh strawberry milkshake made with—			
2% milk	1 cup	121	5
fresh strawberries	1/2 cup	22	0
cinnamon	1/2 tsp.	3	0
Total		*1572 calories*	*45 gm*

25% of total calories from fat

This menu also supplies: 28 gm fiber, 295 mg cholesterol, and 922 mg calcium

7-Day Menu Sampler, continued

Day 2	Serving Size	Calories	Fat (gm)
Breakfast			
grapefruit	1/2	37	0
raisin bran cereal	3/4 cup	131	1
2% milk	1 cup	121	5
Lunch			
Chef's tossed salad made with—			
lettuce	2 cups	20	0
tomato	2 wedges	6	0
sweet green pepper	1/8 pepper	2	0
diced turkey	2 oz.	79	1
shredded mozzarella cheese	1 oz.	79	5
low-fat salad dressing	3 Tbsp.	47	4
whole wheat roll	1	93	2
margarine	1 tsp.	34	4
chilled cantaloupe wedge	1/4 melon	47	0
Dinner			
broiled rib steak	3 oz.	188	9
baked potato	1 medium	220	0
with chives	1 Tbsp.	1	0
low-fat shredded cheddar cheese	1 Tbsp.	12	4
nonfat sour cream	2 tsp.	6	0

7-Day Menu Sampler, continued

Day 2 (continued)	Serving Size	Calories	Fat (gm)
steamed fresh broccoli	3 spears	31	0
with lemon wedge	1/4 lemon	4	0
French bread	1 slice	96	1
margarine	1 tsp.	34	4
fresh fruit medley	3/4 cup	75	0
Snack			
graham cracker	2 squares	59	1
2% milk	1 cup	121	5
Total		*1544 calories*	*44 gm*

25% of total calories from fat

This menu also supplies: 23 gm fiber, 170 mg cholesterol, 1147 mg calcium

7-Day Menu Sampler, continued

Day 3	Serving Size	Calories	Fat (gm)
Breakfast			
chilled orange juice	1/2 cup	54	0
English muffin	1	128	1
low-calorie jam spread	1 tsp.	11	0
2% milk	1 cup	121	5
Lunch			
black bean soup	1 cup	116	1
Swiss cheese	2 oz.	136	10
rye bread	2 slices	130	2
mustard	1 tsp.	4	0
red onion	2 slices	7	0
marinated cucumber salad	4 slices	2	0
with green pepper	1/2 pepper	10	0
low-fat dressing	1 Tbsp.	16	1
green seedless grapes	1 cup	113	1
Dinner			
oven-fried breast of chicken	3 oz.	139	3
made with bread crumbs	2 Tbsp.	49	1
garlic powder	1/2 tsp.	5	0
margarine	1 tsp.	34	4

Day 3 (continued)	Serving Size	Calories	Fat (gm)
Dinner			
pilaf of wild rice	1/2 cup	83	0
stir-fried pea pods	3/4 cup	52	0
spinach salad made with	1 cup spinach	12	0
fresh mushrooms	1/2 cup	9	0
water chestnuts	1/8 cup	16	0
marinated in cider vinegar	1 Tbsp.	2	0
sesame oil	1 tsp.	40	4
soy sauce	3/4 tsp.	2	0
fresh pear slices	1 pear	97	1
Snack			
air-popped popcorn	3 cups	92	1
2% milk	1 cup	121	5
Total		*1601 calories*	*40 gm*

22% of total calories from fat

This menu also supplies: 30 gm fiber, 143 mg cholesterol, 1296 mg calcium

Day 4	Serving Size	Calories	Fat (gm)
Breakfast			
banana	1 medium	104	0
whole wheat bagel	1	143	1
low-calorie jam spread	1 tsp.	10	0
2% milk	1 cup	121	5
Lunch			
salmon croquette made with—			
canned salmon	3 oz.	118	5
bread crumbs	2 Tbsp.	49	1
egg substitute	1 Tbsp.	13	0
chopped onion	1 Tbsp.	4	0
on chopped lettuce	1 cup	7	0
tartar sauce	1 Tbsp.	74	8
fresh carrot	1	31	0
celery sticks	1 stalk	6	0
fresh pineapple chunks	1 cup	76	1

7-Day Menu Sampler, continued

Day 4 (continued)	Serving Size	Calories	Fat (gm)
Dinner			
hamburger	3 oz.	260	11
mixed grain bun	1	118	3
catsup	1 tsp.	5	0
lettuce	2 leaves	5	0
tomato	2 slices	6	0
onion	1 slice	3	0
coleslaw	1/2 cup	89	7
fresh string beans	3/4 cup	33	0
orange sherbet	1/2 cup	132	2
Snack			
apple	1 medium	81	0
2% milk	1 cup	121	5
Total		*1609 calories*	*49 gm*

27% of total calories from fat

This menu also supplies: 22 gm fiber, 131 mg cholesterol, 1133 mg calcium

Day 5	Serving Size	Calories	Fat (gm)
Breakfast			
chilled tomato juice	1/2 cup	21	0
low-cholesterol vegetable omelet made with—			
egg substitute	1/4 cup	52	2
chopped onion	2 Tbsp.	7	0
chopped green pepper	2 Tbsp.	3	0
whole wheat toast	1 slice	80	1
margarine	1 tsp.	34	4
2% milk	1 cup	121	5
Lunch			
black bean soup	1 cup	116	2
cottage cheese	3/4 cup	162	7
stuffed in tomato	1 whole	26	0
sprinkled with paprika	1/8 tsp.	1	0
whole grain crackers	6	140	0
chilled honeydew melon cubes	1 cube	60	0
Dinner			
baked filet of sole	4 oz.	133	2
with bread crumbs	2 Tbsp.	49	1
lemon juice	1 tsp.	1	0
margarine	2 tsp.	68	8

7-Day Menu Sampler, *continued*

Day 5 (continued)	Serving Size	Calories	Fat (gm)
Dinner (continued)			
boiled parsley potatoes	4	84	0
parsley	1/4 tsp.	0	0
squash medley of—			
zucchini	1/4 cup	7	0
summer squash	1/4 cup	9	0
broiled tomato slices	2 slices	13	0
with fresh basil	1/2 tsp.	0	0
angel food cake	1 piece	137	0
with fresh strawberries	1/2 cup	25	0
Snack			
low-fat fruit yogurt	1 cup	250	3
Total		*1599 calories*	*35 gm*

20% of total calories from fat

This menu also supplies: 25 gm fiber, 130 mg cholesterol, 1082 mg calcium

7-Day Menu Sampler, continued

Day 6	Serving Size	Calories	Fat (gm)
Breakfast			
chilled cantaloupe wedge	1/4 melon	49	0
raisin bread	2 slices	137	2
margarine	2 tsp.	68	8
2% milk	1 cup	121	5
Lunch			
Salad Nicoise made with—			
water-packed tuna	3 oz.	98	1
sliced boiled potatoes	2	232	0
fresh green beans	3/4 cup	33	0
ripe olives	5	26	2
hard-cooked egg	1/2	39	3
garbanzo beans	3 tsp.	17	0
tomato	1/2	13	0
lettuce leaves	3	5	0
low-fat salad dressing	3 Tbsp.	47	4
sesame seed crackers	6	91	4
fresh peach slices	1 peach	37	0

7-Day Menu Sampler, continued

Day 6 (continued)	Serving Size	Calories	Fat (gm)
Dinner			
tarragon-roasted chicken breast	3 oz.	139	3
pilaf of brown rice	1/2 cup	108	1
with margarine	1 tsp.	34	4
green peas	1/4 cup	31	0
spring onions	1 tbsp.	2	0
steamed carrots	1/2 cup	35	0
with chopped parsley	1/2 tsp.	0	0
baked apple	1 medium	102	1
with lemon juice	1/2 tsp.	0	0
cinnamon	1/2 tsp.	3	0
Snack			
pretzel sticks	6	11	0
2% milk	1 cup	121	5
Total		*1599 calories*	*43 gm*

24% of total calories from fat

This menu also supplies: 24 gm fiber, 241 mg cholesterol, 892 mg calcium

7-Day Menu Sampler, continued

Day 7	Serving Size	Calories	Fat (gm)
Breakfast			
bran flakes	1 cup	92	0
with banana slices	1 banana	104	0
2% milk	1 cup	121	5
Lunch			
tri-colored pasta salad made with—			
pasta spirals	1 cup cooked	189	1
diced cheddar cheese	2 oz.	227	19
fresh mushrooms	1/8 cup	2	0
fresh broccoli	1/8 cup	3	0
spring onion	2 Tbsp.	4	0
sliced carrots	1/8 cup	6	0
diced red bell pepper	1/8 cup	3	0
lettuce leaves	2	4	0
low-fat salad dressing	2 Tbsp.	31	3
breadsticks	3	115	1
chilled honeydew melon	1/8 melon	90	0

7-Day Menu Sampler, continued

Day 7 (continued)	Serving Size	Calories	Fat (gm)
Dinner			
roasted turkey slices	3 oz.	145	4
baked sweet potato	1 medium	117	0
marinated cucumber salad	1/2 cucumber	20	0
with tomato	1/2 tomato	13	0
low-fat Italian dressing	1 Tbsp.	22	1
whole wheat roll	1	93	2
margarine	1 tsp.	34	4
fresh pineapple chunks	1/2 cup	38	0
Snack			
nonfat frozen yogurt	1/2 cup	103	1
Total		**1576 calories**	**41 gm**

23% of total calories from fat

This menu also supplies: 25 gm fiber, 146 mg cholesterol, 1076 mg calcium

Foods to Stay Vibrant, Young & Healthy

6

Using
Your Nutrition
Label Smarts

E ven though there are obvious links between good nutrition and health, it's not always easy to choose the right foods to keep us healthy. This is partly because many people don't always take time to read and try to understand nutrition labels. Maybe it's because the grocery store is always a madhouse; maybe it's because you are always in a hurry. Whatever the reason, don't be misled by advertising labels on the front of packages. Read the nutrition labels on the back. Here's how.

Did you ever think that a food labeled "low-fat" or "nonfat" was one you could eat in unlimited quantities? Is there a difference between "light" and "lite?" Back in the old days, packaged foods were required only to have their name on the package. But, good news, times have changed, and the growing trend toward health consciousness has led to a new nutrition label, affording the consumer more and better information.

The most recent changes to the food label are the result of the Nutrition Labeling and Education Act, passed by the FDA in 1990 and implemented in May of 1994. The law creates an entirely new food labeling system that appears on virtually all packaged foods. (Exempt foods include food sold by a small business or on site; vending machine foods; coffee, tea, and spices; small packaged items; fresh fruits and vegetables; and raw meat, poultry, and fish.)

The new standards in food labeling provide consumers with more complete, informative, and easy-to-understand facts about individual foods than ever before. "Nutrition Facts" include information on serving sizes, calories, calories from fat, total fat, saturated fat, cholesterol, sodium, complex carbohydrates, dietary fiber, sugar, protein, vitamin A and C, calcium, and iron. Daily values for the nutrients show how the specific food fits into an overall daily diet.

Daily values are based on standard 2000-calorie and 2500-calorie diets. These are used to represent an average for healthy people: 2000 calories for healthy women, young children, or older adults; 2500 calories for men, pregnant women, and teenagers. Now you may not think you eat and drink 2000 calories in a day, but that's the actual average for American women.

Presenting . . . The Food Label

This panel is on almost every food package.

The standard serving size and number of servings in a package are listed here. →

There is no daily value for sugar. Daily values for protein are not required. →

This is found on the bottom of every label. It reminds us how many calories are in one gram of a fat, a carbohydrate, or a protein. →

Nutrition Facts

Serving Size 1/2 cup (114 g)
Servings Per Container 4

Amount Per Serving
Calories 260   Calories from Fat 120

	% Daily Value*
Total Fat 13g	20%
Saturated Fat 5g	25%
Cholesterol 30mg	10%
Sodium 660mg	28%
Total Carbohydrate 31g	11%
Dietary Fiber 0g	0%
Sugars 5g	
Protein 5g	

Vitamin A 4%	•	Vitamin C 2%
Calcium 15%	•	Iron 4%

*Percent Daily Values are based on a 2,000 calorie diet. Your daily values may be higher or lower depending on your calorie needs:

		Calories	2,000	2,500
Total Fat	Less than		65g	80g
Sat Fat	Less than		20g	25g
Cholesterol	Less than		300 mg	300mg
Sodium	Less than		2400mg	2400mg
Total Carbohydrate			300g	375g
Dietary Fiber			25g	30g
Calories per gram:				

Fat 9 • Carbohydrate 4 • Protein 4

Total calories and those calories from fat are listed here. ←

% Daily Values indicates how a serving of this food fits into the overall diet. It is based on a 2000-calorie diet. ←

Other nutrient requirements are listed for both a 2000-calorie and 2500-calorie diet. ←

Let's say, for example, that you're figuring your fat intake. If your break-fast foods make up 40 percent of the recommended daily fat intake, and your lunch adds another 30 percent, you probably won't want to choose foods for dinner that exceed 30 percent. Reading these values off the labels helps you choose foods that add up to, but don't go over, the recommended total daily intake.

At the bottom of the label, the total recommended daily values appear (not just the percentages) for other nutrients so you can get an idea of the total amounts required. Use these figures as your guide when you select foods to fit into your personal daily foodstyle.

One Size Fits All

Have you ever checked the nutrition label on a bag of potato chips and been amazed at how low in fat they are? Pay attention to how fast that happy feeling disappears when you discover that a serving size is just three tiny chips. As if anyone could stop eating them after only three chips! Luckily, with the new food labels, this kind of surprise should not occur. No more can one brand of macaroni and cheese say one serving is equivalent to 3/4 cup while another brand says one serving is 1/2 cup. Now, all similar foods must follow the same serving size requirements. This lets you compare similar products without having to do a lot of mental arithmetic.

It's What's Inside That Counts

The most important thing you can do is read a product's list of ingredients. Reading the fine print tells the truth about the contents of the package. The ingredient list can help you avoid foods that you're allergic to or that your body can't process. Ingredients are listed in order, and the ingredient present in the largest amount by weight is listed first. Other ingredients are listed in descending order according to weight.

Additives must also be listed, and if artificial colors are used, the manufacturer must list FDA-certified color additives by name. Colors exempt from certification, such as caramel, paprika, and beet juice, can simply be named as "artificial colors."

Products with "standards of identity," which meant their recipes were defined by law, used to be able to omit an ingredient list. Today even they are subject to the new food labeling law. You will now find an ingredient list on such things as catsup, macaroni, jelly, and orange juice.

Getting What You Pay For

Often the size of a package can be deceiving. There are few of us who haven't opened a bag of pretzels only to find it half filled with air. Always look at the package weight. A large box or package may contain less product by weight than a smaller package. The weight should be listed in both ounce or pound units and metric units. Remember, it's the weight of the package, not the size of the box, that matters. Good things can still come in small packages when it comes to food.

Wanted: A Date

Product dates are used to give you an idea of how long a product will remain fresh and healthy. Product dating and the wording used are regulated by the FDA. Some common product dates are:

Pull date—
This date shows how long the manufacturer thinks a product should stay on the grocery shelves. Appearing on a label as "Sell by" or "Best when purchased by," these dates take into account time for home storage and consumption. They are calculated by the manufacturer, based on knowledge of the product and the product's shelf life.

Quality assurance or freshness date—

This date shows when the quality of a product is not at its best. On the label, it appears after "Best if used by. . . ." While the product might not taste as good after the freshness date, it doesn't mean there's anything nutritionally wrong with it.

Expiration date—

This date, which usually appears after "Use by" or "Do not use after," gives you the last day on which a product should be eaten. State governments regulate these dates for perishable items.

Sticker Shock

Supermarkets that display unit prices make it easy for you to compare prices. Unit prices are found on stickers, usually located on the edge of the shelf below the food item. Unit pricing helps you pick the least expensive package or container size and helps you compare prices of similar packages.

The unit price label will show you:

- brand name
- description of product
- size of package
- retail price (the price of the package as a whole)
- unit price (the price per ounce, pound, pint, quart, or number of items in a package)

Who's Responsible For This?

Food labels must list the company responsible for the product—whether it's the manufacturer, packer, or distributor—and the company's city, state, and zip code. If you find something wrong with a product, you shouldn't hesitate to let the company know.

What Do All Those Terms Mean?

Certain terms have become so common that it's hard to tell what they really mean. New strict labeling laws and definitions have been set by the FDA and must be followed by manufacturers. Here's a rundown of what various claims mean:

Reduced, Less, Fewer—
These apply to foods that have been altered to contain at least 25 percent less of whatever it is that's reduced. For example, a package might say "Reduced Fat," "Less Sodium," or "Fewer Calories." The claim must include the percent of difference and the name of the product it's being compared to. If the regular product already meets "low" standards, the new product can't make "reduced" claims.

Lite, Light—
These apply to foods that contain at least one-third less calories or 50 percent less fat than the regular product. It can also mean foods that have half the sodium content of the reference product. Other references to lite or light can refer to color, breading, or texture, but this should be noted on the label.

High, Rich in, Excellent Source—
These terms refer to foods containing 20 percent or more of the Daily Value for that nutrient in a serving. For example, "High in Fiber," "Rich in Protein," or "Excellent Source of Calcium."

Good Source, Contains, Provides—
These can be stated on a label if a food contains 11 to 19 percent more of the Daily Value for the specific nutrient in a serving. For example, "Good Source of Iron," "Contains Fiber," or "Provides Vitamin C."

More—
This refers to any food that has 10 percent more than the Daily Value per serving of a specific nutrient compared to the regular product. Dissimilar products can also be compared, such as frozen yogurt and ice cream.

Free—

Products that say this have insignificant amounts of calories, fat, saturated fat, cholesterol, sodium, and/or sugar. Other synonyms for the term "free" are "No," "Zero," "Negligible source of," "Dietarily insignificant source of," or "Without." Examples are:

- *Calorie Free*—must contain less than 5 calories per serving

- *Cholesterol Free*—must have less than 2 milligrams of cholesterol and 2 grams or less of saturated fat per serving.

- *Fat Free*—contains less than 0.5 grams of fat per serving

- *Sugar Free*—must have less than 0.5 grams of sugar per serving.

Low, Little, Few—

These refer to products that don't exceed dietary guidelines for calories, fat, saturated fat, cholesterol, and/or sodium. Examples are:

- *Low Fat*—contains 3 grams or less per serving
- *Low Saturated Fat*—has 1 gram or less per serving, with no more than 15 percent of calories per serving coming from saturated fat
- *Low Sodium*—contains 140 milligrams or less per serving

- *Very Low Sodium*—has 35 milligrams or less per serving

- *Low Cholesterol*—contains 20 milligrams or less per serving

- *Low Calorie*—has 40 calories or less per serving

Lean, Extra Lean—

These apply to the fat content of meats, poultry, and seafood or fish. Examples are:

- *Lean*—contains less than 10 grams of fat, less than 4 grams of saturated fat, and less than 95 milligrams of cholesterol per serving.

- *Extra Lean*—has less than 5 grams of fat, less than 2 grams of saturated fat, and less than 95 milligrams of cholesterol per serving (per 100 grams of the product's weight).

Enriched, Fortified—
These apply to foods that have been nutritionally altered to increase the Daily Value of one or more nutrients by at least 10 percent.

Percent Fat Free—
Foods with this claim must meet the standards for low fat since people assume they can be included in a low-fat diet. The claim must also reflect the amount of fat present in 100 grams of the food. For example, if a food contains 3 grams of fat per 75 grams, it's "96-percent fat free." But if a product states that it is "85% Fat Free," it may be more revealing to look at the calories from fat and the total fat grams.

Claims About Nutrition and Diseases

It should be obvious to all of us that what we eat has a vital effect on our overall health. Foods definitely impact our health and well-being. In some cases, food labels carry information relating to current health issues, such as eating too much fat, saturated fat, and cholesterol, but not enough fruits, vegetables, and high-fiber foods, and the relationship between this pattern and heart disease or certain kinds of cancer. While this information may be useful, other factors are at play, besides diet, such as genetics and exercise, when it comes to your susceptibility to these diseases.

Health claims that the FDA allows on product packages include:

Calcium and Osteoporosis—
Having a diet low in calcium is one risk factor for osteoporosis, a disease that causes lowered bone mass, particularly in women. Getting adequate amounts of calcium can help bones develop properly in the teen years and can help slow the rate of bone loss later in life. Foods that claim high calcium and link osteoporosis to calcium must have:

—at least 200 milligrams of calcium

—no more phosphorous than calcium per serving

—calcium in an easily absorbed state

Fat and Cancer —

Diets low in fat have been shown to reduce the risk of some types of cancer, such as breast cancer, colon cancer, and prostate cancer. While doctors and scientists don't know why this is true, the incidence of these cancers is higher among those who consume diets high in fat. A diet that is made up of 30 percent or less of calories from fat is recommended. To claim this relationship, a food must have:

—3 grams or less of fat per serving

—5 grams or less of fat per serving for fish or game meats, the "Extra Lean" requirement

Saturated Fat, Cholesterol, and Coronary Heart Disease—

Diets high in saturated fat and cholesterol are known to increase LDL blood cholesterol levels and thereby increase the risk of coronary heart disease. Diets low in saturated fat and cholesterol can decrease this risk. To make this claim, foods must contain:

—3 grams or less of fat per serving

—20 milligrams of cholesterol or less per serving

—1 gram or less of saturated fat per serving

—5 grams or less of fat per serving for fish or game meats, the "Extra Lean" requirement

Fiber-Rich Grain Products, Fruits, Vegetables, and Cancer—

Diets high in fiber and low in fat and cholesterol can reduce the risk of some forms of cancer. This is a fact even though it is not totally understood why. Food products making this claim must contain:

—a grain, fruit, or vegetable

—3 grams or less of fat per serving

—at least 2 grams of dietary fiber

Fiber-Rich Grain Products, Fruits, Vegetables, and Heart Disease—
Diets high in fiber and low in fat and cholesterol are known to reduce blood cholesterol levels, thus reducing the risk of heart disease. To make this claim, products must have:

—a grain, fruit, or vegetable

—3 grams or less of fat per serving

—less than 20 milligrams of cholesterol per serving

—1 gram or less of saturated fat per serving (15 percent or less of calories from saturated fat)

—0.6 grams or more of soluble dietary fiber per serving

Sodium and High Blood Pressure—
Low sodium diets may help reduce the incidence of hypertension (high blood pressure), which is a risk factor for coronary heart disease and strokes. To claim this relationship, a food product must contain:

—140 milligrams or less of sodium per serving

Fruits, Vegetables, and Cancer—
Diets that are high in fruits and vegetables, and low in fat, may lead to a reduced risk of cancer, but once again it's not completely understood why. To apply this claim, a food must have:

—a fruit or vegetable

—3 grams or less of fat per serving

—at least 500 IU (International Units) of vitamin A, 6 milligrams of vitamin C, or 2.5 grams of dietary fiber per serving

Don't let this labeling information overwhelm you. We know it can be confusing, but, while you don't need to memorize any of it, you may want to know how to use it in your personal foodstyle. Putting this information to work for you at the grocery store can make a world of difference. You should also find it reassuring that the FDA and food manufacturers are finally responding to consumer demand for more accurate and adequate information about the foods we eat.

7
Grocery Shopping:
Grueling Grind or
Fast and Fun?

It probably won't surprise you to learn that most of us buy the same 20 foods every time we grocery shop. We get into a rut. Tired of wandering the cereal lane for the hundredth time, we become afflicted with that dreaded energy-sucking disease—supermarket fatigue!

Wouldn't it be nice to add a little variety to your life? Spice it up! Vibrant, young, and healthy shoppers take some chances. They try new and daring things. Sure, this could mean wearing a costume when you shop. Or, it could mean in-line skating down the aisles behind your cart. But, what we recommend is trying new foods; add at least one new food to your shopping list and your healthy life each week.

You probably go to the store intending to buy only what your family needs. But, once you're there, the temptations of the supermarket can lure you in many different directions. You may buy foods you don't really want, need, or even like! Sometimes, we buy things that are on sale for that sole reason: they are on sale!

Vitamin C-rich foods are thought to prevent atherosclerosis, so try to eat more citrus fruits, strawberries, tomatoes, broccoli, dark-green, leafy vegetables, sweet potatoes, and cantaloupe.

Have you noticed that staple food items are always displayed along the sides and back of the store? This is specifically designed to make you walk through the aisles so you'll be enticed into making purchases along the way—whether or not you need any of these things. How can you get control?

Planning is the key to efficient and pleasurable grocery shopping. Make a list and clip coupons, only for items you really need and normally use, of course. It's a good idea to shop after you've eaten since when you're less hungry, you're less likely to be tempted by hollow-calorie foods that offer nothing but instant and short-term gratification. And remember, a bargain is only a bargain if it's something you really need. A coupon can be worthless if a store-brand or generic-brand item is less expensive and just as good.

Productive Purchasing Practices in Produce

There are no foodstyle "bad guys" in the produce department because most fruits and vegetables are high in fiber, naturally low in sodium, and, with the exception of avocados and nuts, most contain virtually no fat. Fruits and vegetables have no cholesterol and many are low in calories, too. Needless to say, fruits and vegetables are great vibrant, young, and healthy foodstyle choices.

One cup of parsley provides an entire day's supply of vitamins A, C and iron. This natural breath freshener is being studied for its cancer-preventing benefits.

Fresh fruits and vegetables in their season are almost always less expensive than their canned or frozen counterparts. Look for apples in the winter, tomatoes and melons in the summer, fresh peaches and strawberries in the spring, and pumpkins and grapes in the fall.

Vitamins A, C, E, and the mineral selenium are believed to be important for their "antioxidant" qualities. Oxidation plays a role in aging, according to some researchers. They claim eating foods rich in antioxidants slows the aging process and can be effective in keeping body cells healthy.

Choose deep green or yellow fruits and vegetables for more vitamin A. Romaine lettuce, raw spinach, and green leaf lettuce are better salad choices than iceberg lettuce, which is mainly water and lower in vitamins. Acorn squash, carrots, apricots, cantaloupe, and broccoli are highly nutritious choices, too.

If it's vitamin C you're after, you don't have to settle only for orange juice. Raw green peppers, sliced tomatoes, broccoli, raw cabbage, potatoes, and strawberries are all rich in vitamin C. Vitamin E is also present in broccoli, peaches, dried prunes, asparagus, avocados, and spinach. Selenium, a mineral important in healthy living, is found in most vegetables grown in the ground. The amount of selenium found in food depends on the condition of the soil in which it is grown.

Be careful in the produce section, however, and stick to your list. Often we tend to buy more than our household can eat before the fresh foods spoil. Brown bananas are not attractive on the kitchen counter, are they? Look for smaller packages of vegetables if you know you can't eat that whole head of lettuce or pound of carrots. Prewashed salad mixes are packed airtight, come in variously sized packages, and are perfect for busy women who still want fresh vegetables for their families. More and more grocers are getting the message and are packing smaller portions of raw vegetables. Some produce even comes conveniently grated or sliced.

Plan to eat some of your vegetables raw today and then steam them for tomorrow night's meal. Since many fruits, especially berries, are highly perishable, use them quickly or freeze them for later use. And, if you want just enough salad for one meal, head for the supermarket salad bar.

Step Up to the Salad Bar

It's not a bad idea to take a good look at everything on a salad bar before you dig in. Make sure everything is fresh and then choose only the freshest items. Fill your container with foods you wouldn't ordinarily buy in bulk. The salad bar is a great way to try something new. Be careful to avoid those mixed salads made with mayonnaise or oils, however, since they are loaded with hidden fat, no matter how tasty and tempting they look.

Making the Most of the Meat Counter

Ask your butcher about the leanest cut of meat available. Even though it may be a little more expensive, trust us, it's worth it.

Lean beef, pork, lamb, and ham may not be much different in price than fish or chicken, but they often contain more fat . . . and most of it is saturated. Look for lean, well trimmed cuts such as flank, round, sirloin, or tenderloin steaks, pork tenderloin, and lean ham. The new lean pork is as lean as chicken. Meats graded "select" are leaner than those graded "choice." Buy skinless chicken or remove the skin before you cook it. Most of the fat in chicken lies just beneath the skin.

Freshly ground turkey is low in fat, but be aware that many of the frozen varieties contain up to 15 percent turkey skin that's not listed on the label. You may prefer to grind your own skinless turkey or chop it in the food processor. Many fresh cuts of turkey, such as turkey steaks and turkey medallions, are available nowadays and they make good lean foodstyle choices.

Buy only one-fourth pound of boneless trimmed meat, poultry, or fish per person. Meat, fish, and poultry shrink about 25 percent during cooking, so 4 ounces of raw meat equals about 3 ounces of cooked meat, just the right size for a serving. The following raw portions equal 3 ounces of cooked meat:

- 1/4 pound ground beef
- One side (half) of a chicken breast
- One chicken leg and thigh
- 1/2 Rock Cornish game hen
- One 3x3-inch piece of fish, 3/4-inch thick

Any kind of fish fillet is a good choice because fish is easy to cook and to digest. Salmon and

Oils contain no water and are 100 percent fat! They do vary, however, in the amount of saturated fat they contain.

~

other cold-water fish, such as tuna, mackerel, sea trout, and herring, are heart-healthy selections. Don't buy fish that has been previously frozen if you plan to refreeze it. Repeated thawing can cause increased bacterial growth and diminished taste and texture in fish. Cook previously frozen, thawed fish soon after purchase.

Diving into the Dairy Case

Cheddar cheese is very high in fat as are many varieties of cheese. You can make the cheese you use go farther by buying sharp or extra sharp flavors. With their stronger taste, you don't need to use as much to flavor your dishes. Many new reduced-fat cheddar-type cheeses still have good flavor. Serve them at room temperature for the best taste.

Try string cheese, part-skim ricotta, and some of the new low-fat natural cheeses for a lower fat foodstyle. You can also opt for cheese made with skim milk, 1% milk, or buttermilk, or for low-fat cottage cheese or nonfat yogurt. They offer all the nutrition but less fat than traditional products.

When you buy margarine, choose brands that have the least amount of saturated fat. Remember to read labels. The amount of saturated fat is listed on the nutrition label. Most margarines contain 1 to 2 grams of saturated fat. Tub margarines are generally better for you than sticks. Liquid oil should always be listed as the first ingredient. Water content varies among margarines and calories will vary from 50 to 100 per tablespoon among spreads, whipped, and regular margarine styles. Regular butter contains about 100 calories per tablespoon.

Cook oatmeal in part low-fat milk and part water to boost calcium content.

There is still controversy about margarine because of how it is processed from an oil into hydrogenated fat. It's best to use as little margarine as possible, regardless of how it's made, since only one tablespoon of regular margarine a day (at 100 calories per tablespoon) above your needs equals a weight gain of 10 pounds in one year.

Eggs should always be stored at 45 degrees Fahrenheit or colder, so check out the refrigeration at the store. Eggs stored at a higher temperature have a greater chance of being infected with the bacteria salmonella. Egg substitutes are a good option for lower fat and cholesterol foodstyles.

Deliberating at the Deli Counter

Sliced or shaved turkey, smoked turkey, and lean roast beef are good choices among low-fat cold cuts. Yes, they are more expensive than cooking the meat yourself, but the convenience of buying just what you need is worth the extra expense to many busy women. Use deli meats within 2 or 3 days. You can always divide larger packages of deli meats into 2-ounce portions and freeze them for later use. Canadian bacon and lean ham can also be part of a healthy foodstyle, but they are high in sodium. If you are concerned about your salt intake, choose a lower-salt deli meat.

Many cold cuts and lunch meats are not bargains, so be careful. It's a good idea to figure out the price per pound, not just the price per package. You may learn that you've been paying an exorbitant amount for bologna! Lean boiled ham and turkey cold cuts can be low in fat, but compare their fat content to the amount of fat in an ounce of freshly baked turkey on the following chart.

Decrease the salt in your recipes and substitute a variety of spices and herbs for flavor. Light-seasoned salt has less sodium than regular salt. Use garlic and onion powders instead of garlic and onion salt. Remember, one teaspoon of salt has about 2000 milligrams of sodium.

How Much Fat in Cold Cuts?

Food Item (1 oz.)	Approximate Grams of Fat per Serving
baked turkey, light meat	1
baked turkey, dark meat	2
turkey bologna	5
turkey salami	3 to 4
turkey hot dog	4 to 11
turkey ham	1.5
turkey pastrami	1
boiled ham	1.4
bologna	8 to 10
hot dog	8 to 17
salami	8 to 17
pastrami	8 to 10

Note: The fat content in cold cuts varies from brand to brand, so be sure to read the labels.

Browsing the Bread and Cereal Shelves

These days more and more women are jumping on the "bran wagon." If you are among them, you should look for whole grain breads and cereals that say "100% whole wheat" on the label. Some breads contain caramel color instead of whole grains.

Whole wheat flour or whole cracked wheat should be listed as the first ingredient on the label when you select your bread or cereal. Wheat flour, unbleached wheat flour, and enriched wheat flour are all really just white flour. If the label lists whole wheat flour as the first ingredient and enriched wheat flour as the second or third ingredient, then the bread still contains at least 50 percent whole wheat flour.

Most bread is low in fat and shouldn't contain more than 1 gram of fat per slice. But be careful: soft dinner rolls, croissants, and canned rolls and biscuits do contain more fat. Read the label.

Bagels, pita bread, English muffins, corn tortillas, and French bread are most often made with flour, yeast, and salt. They usually don't contain fats, oils, eggs, or sugar, but you should check the label to make sure. Cinnamon raisin and garlic bagels can be a tasty change of pace. Slice the bagels in half before you stick them in the freezer so all you have to do is pop them in the toaster when you feel like having them.

Calcium not only reduces the risk of osteo-porosis, it also is an important regulator of blood pressure and heart function.

Check crackers for ingredients because they often contain hidden fat. Most popular brands used to contain coconut oil and palm oil, but many manufacturers have switched to vegetable oil and reduced the fat content. Some crackers, like crispbreads and flatbreads, are particularly low in fat and make a good healthy foodstyle choice.

You know, you can make your own chips from corn tortillas or pita bread. Just spray the tortillas with vegetable cooking spray and sprinkle them with paprika, garlic powder, chili powder, and cumin. Cut them into wedges and bake at 350° until they are crisp. Let them cool and then eat and enjoy! You've created a low-calorie, low-in-fat healthy snack. New, baked chips also are available in stores. They're convenient but expensive.

Thick pretzels are another good low-in-fat snack. Just be sure to rub off the extra salt before you eat them.

> *Tofu, or soybean curd, is great source of protein and calcium and low in cholesterol and calorie—an excellent substitute for meats.*

If you are looking for a good source of fiber, select cereals with fiber content readings of 4 grams or more per serving. Fortified cereals and those labeled multi-vitamin supplements have extra vitamins and minerals. If you select one of these cereals, you may not need to take that vitamin or mineral supplement, depending on your body's needs. Look for cereals with 5 grams or less of sugar and 2 grams or less of fat per serving.

Figuring Out the Frozen Food Case

Plain vegetables, frozen right after they've been harvested, are champions when it comes to nutrition. They have no added fat and less salt than vegetables in sauce. Use a bag of frozen vegetables and you pour out just what you need for each meal. Reseal the bag and put it back in the freezer.

Frozen concentrate is usually the most economical form of fruit juice to buy. Fruit beverages in boxes or pouches contain more water and sugar than real fruit juice, so be wary when you use them.

For breakfast, frozen waffles and pancakes can be quick and convenient, and many of these products are made with some whole grain. Check the label to find out exactly what you're eating.

Many people find it hard to live without a daily "fix" of ice cream. When shopping for frozen desserts, compare the fat content of deluxe ice creams, regular ice creams, ice milk, and frozen yogurt products. Ice milk and frozen yogurt products should have less fat, but sometimes they have almost as many calories because of their higher sugar content. Sugar-free desserts still have some calories and often some fat. A 100-calorie limit of these low-calorie products can fit into most low-calorie foodstyles.

Food for Thought: Frozen Dinners

Frozen dinners are here to stay, and they are actually getting better. It's still important to be careful when making your frozen entree choice, however. Nutritionally, some of these meals sink whereas others swim.

It's no wonder that frozen dinner sales have soared to more than $1 billion annually. They're convenient and they're great for single or busy women who don't count cooking as one of their favorite activities. Frozen dinners are also affordable—often costing less than a fast-food meal—and they're as close as your freezer. You can store them for up to one year. There are as many varieties to choose from as your moods dictate: from meatloaf to manicotti.

Many frozen dinners have evolved from mundane and bland to tasty, calorie-controlled, gourmet-style meals. When choosing frozen dinners, consider the following as a guide for getting the best product for your needs:

- Look for nutritional content as well as calorie content.

- Look for frozen entrees with a protein content of at least 10 to 15 grams.

- Even if you are restricting your calories, you should eat about 300 to 500 calories at your main meal. (This is usually dinner for today's active women.) Many of the low-calorie dinners contain less than 300 calories—and that's not enough for most women. These dinners are not nutritionally complete by themselves and should be supplemented. You need something to go with them, like salad and/or fruit, to nutritionally round them out.

> *You can't go wrong with the high-nutrition, low-calorie cantaloupe. Half a melon supplies more than 150% of the daily requirements of vitamin C, more than 800 mg of potassium, and 100% of the requirement for beta carotene.*

- Most frozen dinners don't provide much fiber. Be sure to eat whole grain breads, high-fiber cereals, and additional fruits, vegetables, and legumes at other meals.

- Many frozen dinners are high in sodium, so if you're watching your salt intake, be sure to read the labels and choose the lower sodium varieties.

- Except for a very few entrees, frozen dinners usually aren't a primary source of calcium. Include high-calcium foods, such as milk, in your dinner or drink some milk at some time during your day.

- If you shop for low-fat frozen dinners, try to select those with less than 10 grams of fat. Eating a low-fat frozen entree allows room for some extra fat like salad dressing or margarine on a roll. Remember, it's your overall fat intake in a day that's important, not just the fat in a specific food.

- Always look at the servings per package on frozen entrees. Most are only one serving. Some, however, say they contain two servings, even though one person could easily finish the whole container.

For example, we went to the grocery store and did a little comparison shopping, not in price per pound, but in nutrition value per frozen dinner. Here's what we found:

Look at the nutrition values for a *Banquet® Meat Loaf Dinner, Extra Helping* size (but intended to serve one person):

Calories	650
Calories from fat	340
Total fat	38 gm
Cholesterol	85 mg
Sodium	2100 mg

Compare that with a *Regular Swanson's® Meat Loaf Dinner* for one:

Calories	410
Calories from fat	160
Total Fat	18 gm
Cholesterol	35 mg
Sodium	1060 mg

Compare both with a *Healthy Choice® Meat Loaf Dinner* for one:

Calories	320
Calories from fat	80
Total Fat	8 gm
Cholesterol	35 mg
Sodium	460 mg

Or a *Stouffer's Lean Cuisine® Meat Loaf Dinner* for one:

Calories	270
Calories from fat	81
Total Fat	9 gm
Cholesterol	55 mg
Sodium	540 mg

And finally, here's a *Stouffer's® regular Meat Loaf Dinner* for one:

Calories	390
Calories from Fat	210
Total Fat	24 gm
Cholesterol	80 mg
Sodium	910 mg

To make a really accurate comparison, you'd want to look at the actual size of the serving to see how many ounces it totals. Then compare serving size for serving size. Now, we think most women don't have time for this, so they'll check out the values that we listed on page 149.

It seems obvious that when you have an opportunity to choose, assuming that all offerings have at least a reasonable amount of flavor or they wouldn't even be in the market, you'd probably opt for the least amount of fat, right? Well, then, how about calories? Maybe sodium? Whatever your criteria, choose the one that fits best into your healthy foodstyle.

Here's another comparison, this time of chicken entrees.

Banquet® BBQ Chicken Meal (for one):

Calories	320
Calories from fat	110
Total fat	12 gm
Cholesterol	60 mg
Sodium	800 mg

Compare that with *Swanson's® Chicken Nuggets*:

Calories	500
Calories from fat	220
Total fat	24 gm
Cholesterol	50 mg
Sodium	720 mg

Now look at *Healthy Choice® Country Herb Chicken*:

Calories	270
Calories from fat	35
Total fat	4 gm

Cholesterol	35 mg
Sodium	340 mg

Or with *Stouffer's Lean Cuisine® Herb Roasted Chicken:*

Calories	210
Calories from fat	40
Total fat	5 gm
Cholesterol	40 mg
Sodium	430 mg

Look at these values to determine which one you would choose and think about for what reasons you'd choose it. If your guidelines are based on lowered calories and lowered fat, you're on your way to a healthy foodstyle. Here's our list of other frozen dinners that fit well into the healthy foodstyle:

And the Winners Are. . .

Le Menu Lite® —
Turkey Divan
Chicken Cacciatore
Herb Roasted Chicken

Stouffer's Lean Cuisine®—
Chicken Marsala
Glazed Chicken with Vegetables
Turkey Breast

Weight Watchers®—
Chicken Fajitas
London Broil

And, any Healthy Choice® dinner.

Contemplating Canned Foods

Many stores typically place name brand items at eye level, but good buys can be found by looking for generic or store brands on lower or higher shelves. Most brands have exactly the same nutritional values and taste just as good as nationally advertised brands. But they can cost half as much.

Most canned fruits and vegetables are quality foods because they are canned at the peak of their ripeness. But, since salt is used as a preservative in canning, some may have a higher salt content than others. Many manufacturers are trying to lower the salt content of their canned foods, and many low-salt options are becoming available. For their convenience and economy, canned foods can certainly have a place in your foodstyle.

Canned fruits, for example, are a staple in many homes. If this is true for you, look for fruit packed in juice rather than in heavy syrup to keep calories in check.

Look for evaporated skim milk or nonfat dry milk. These can be used as coffee lighteners and are a good source of calcium. Dry nondairy creamers contain mostly saturated fat and sugar and have no calcium at all. The latter have no benefit in any foodstyle.

Thin out thick, creamy dressings with buttermilk, plain yogurt, or low-fat milk.

~

Stock up on kidney beans, pinto beans, and lentils; they're a quick and easy source of dietary fiber, and canned varieties take only minutes to prepare.

Fats, Oils, and Salad Dressings

All oils, except palm and coconut oil, consist primarily of unsaturated fat. Canola, rapeseed, and safflower oils contain the least amount of saturated fat. Some oils have the word "light" on their label, but that may refer to color instead of calories or fat content, so beware! "Light" mayonnaise has half the calories of regular mayonnaise and is still quite tasty.

Bottled dressings may be low in calories, but not low in salt. You can make your own low-calorie dressing by thinning creamy dressings with non-fat yogurt or light mayonnaise. Low calorie dressings are great not only on salads but also as marinades for poultry, meat, and vegetables.

Ripe olives are fairly low in calories but are high in both fat and salt. Five medium olives contain 45 calories and the equivalent of one teaspoon of fat. Use all peanut butter sparingly. Two teaspoons equal one teaspoon of fat and one tablespoon has over 100 calories.

> *Use reduced-calorie mayonnaise and salad dressings to lower both fat and calories in your recipes. Don't pour. Dribble salad dressing over salad. Or better yet, measure out dressing and toss in bowl before serving.*

Picking Packaged Cookies and Snacks

Good cookie choices are gingersnaps, fig bars, vanilla wafers, and graham crackers. Cookies labeled fat-free or low-fat, as well as some oatmeal cookies and cookies made with cocoa, are good choices for a low-in-fat foodstyle as long as you stick to the serving size noted on the package. The best way to find out if cookies are low in fat and calories is to check the label.

Even potato and corn chips can be found today in low-fat and fat-free versions. Let your taste buds determine which you prefer, but remember that these still contain calories, so don't eat the entire bag in one sitting. Rice cakes and popcorn cakes are also available in a variety of sizes and flavors. They are a tasty, healthy choice for snacking. While the taste and texture may not appeal to you at first, take a chance. Be daring. They might grow on you.

Air-popped popcorn is the lowest calorie popcorn, and is the best among the best of the low-calorie, low-fat snack choices. If you sprinkle it with butter-flavored granules, you get most of the flavor without any of the fat of real butter. Packaged and microwave popcorns (even the low-fat and light varieties) can contain over double the calories and as much fat as corn chips or even potato chips, so read labels. It's often high in saturated fat, too. If you don't have an air-popper machine, pop your own in a small amount of vegetable oil. Or look for microwave varieties with less than 3 grams of fat per serving. Compare popcorn with the other snacks on the chart below.

Snack Chart

Food	Serving Size	Calories
popcorn, air popped	1 cup	20
popcorn, old fashioned popper with oil	1 cup	40
popcorn, microwave variety	1 cup	45 to 65
pretzels	1 ring	11
corn chips	1	4
potato chips	1 chip	12
rice cakes	1 mini cake	10

Checking Out

Once you reach the checkout counter, you might want to spend your time in line looking over your selections instead of sneaking a peak at the tempting tabloids. Look in your cart. Did you pick a variety of foods? Did you remember to try at least one new food this week? Did you get enough food for yourself or your entire family? Did you get too much?

Remember, you don't have to cut out all the foods you love to eat when you move toward a healthy foodstyle. With planning, watching your food intake can be as easy as adding a little spice to your life. Try out new foods and don't be afraid to experiment. If in-line skating through the aisles still sounds like more fun, check with your grocer—then go for it. We told you, grocery shopping can be fast and fun!

8

Dining In, Dining Out, Dining Meatless

Don't you like the word, dining? It makes us think of an elegant event: something refined, something leisurely. Dining with friends; dining out; dining at Le Cafe du Monde—it all evokes something pleasant, doesn't it?

Well, lots of us eat out these days. But what a difference between "dining out" and "eating out." When we approach the midlife years, we should really be striving for more dining and less eating.

Throughout history, dining has been recognized as one of humankind's great pleasures. The Romans did it lying down. Europeans still do it with style—late at night in the Mediterranean countries, lingering for hours in Italy, and enjoying course after course with just the right wine in France.

Wherever we dine, out on the town or at home, women all over the western world are becoming concerned about dining on the right foods and feeling good. In this chapter, we learn how to make the right choices to fit a vibrant, young, and healthy foodstyle.

Dining Out

Garlic contains cancer-preventing properties and may reduce heart attacks and stroke by preventing clumping of blood cells that lead to clots. A half clove of fresh garlic daily is suggested.

~

"Eating out" has become a regular part of daily life for today's active women and their families. And yes, it can be incorporated into a healthy foodstyle, provided you watch portion sizes and selections. While we all love to get our money's worth, many restaurants serve portions more sized to the active, 6-foot 5-inch lumberjack than for today's woman. Being aware of this simple fact can help you adopt a healthy "dining-out" attitude for your personal foodstyle.

Make it your policy to frequent only those restaurants known for their quality cuisine. Many modern chefs are just as health-conscious as we are, so many restaurants are serving lighter, leaner fare. Their menus offer healthy options for patrons who are watching their calories and/or fat intake. And, if you ask, most fine restaurants will alter your food to suit your needs. It's that simple: just ask.

Tips for Dining Out

- Don't starve yourself all day to make room for a hearty dinner. You'll be too hungry and you won't really enjoy the food at all.

- Select full service restaurants (over fast food) offering a variety of choices.

- Avoid high-calorie, high-fat meals. That means to steer clear of certain food preparation techniques. We've listed them along with their definitions so you can understand why these are not in the best interest of anyone pursuing the healthy foodstyle.

A la mode —with ice cream

Au Fromage—with cheese

Au Gratin— in a cheese sauce

Au Lait—with milk

Basted—with added fat

Bisque—a cream soup

Creamed—fat has been added

Crispy—it's fried

Escalloped—with cream sauce

Fried or pan fried—with added fat

Hash—there's added fat

Hollandaise—with cream sauce

Sauteed—there's added fat

- Remove optional foods from the table. They are tempting and distract you from the main meal. Bread baskets, tortilla chips, and crackers are usually eaten just because they are there, not because you are even really interested in them. Ask your server to take them away.

- Eat slowly and enjoy your meal. That's what "dining" is all about. If you want to eat light, choose soup and/or salad, or use the appetizer menu for your choice of entree.

Making Healthy Choices

Always check the menu for items flagged as having less fat or calories. Special symbols are sometimes used to identify lighter fare. Some restaurants offer portions in two sizes—one for the hearty appetite and one for calorie-conscious customers. Sometimes there are even smaller portions on the children's menu that can be made available for adults.

Order foods that are grilled, baked, broiled, steamed, or poached instead of those dipped in heavy batter and fried. Avoid creamed, scalloped, or buttered items. They are high in fat and in calories. Order a la carte. You don't have to have a seven-course meal to enjoy dining out.

Try ordering an appetizer or a luncheon-sized portion as your main dinner course; the serving size will be smaller. Or ask to split entrees and salads. If these options are not available, consider dividing your entree portion in half, eating only half, and boxing the remainder to take home for another day.

Use 1/3 cup oil when recipes call for 1/2 cup butter or shortening.

How about eating your bread without butter, the way they do in Europe? You may find you really enjoy the true taste of bread if it isn't smeared with all that fat.

A good server will be happy to answer your questions about the menu, tell you what ingredients are in each dish, and describe each cooking style.

Ask to have sauces and salad dressings served on the side so that you are in control of how much you eat. These extras are the hidden sources of calories and fat and can ruin your foodstyle day. Remember, two tablespoons of bleu cheese or oil and vinegar salad dressing contain 140 to 160 calories. Two tablespoons of bearnaise or hollandaise sauce contain 110 calories.

Use applesauce in place of half of the fat in recipes. When 1/2 cup margarine is called for, use 1/4 cup margarine and 1/4 cup applesauce.

Avoid buffets or smorgasbords offering all-you-can-eat meals. Few of us have the willpower to stop with small servings of a few foods when a large variety is there for the tasting. On the other hand, a cafeteria can be a good place to take control and choose foods that best fit into your daily foodstyle. Although you won't always know just how much fat has been used in cooking or how much salt has been added, you can, just by looking, get a pretty good idea of how the food is prepared, what the ingredients are, and how large the portion is.

Remember, a drink adds calories. Order your cocktail mixed with water or soda rather than a presweetened mix. How about trying the refreshing taste of calorie-free sparkling water with lemon or lime?

Lower-fat Menu Choices for Dining Out

- When selecting soup, order consomme, broth, vegetable soup, minestrone, gazpacho, or any other clear soup.

- In the appetizer category, try fruit cups, smoked salmon, crudites, or broiled mushrooms, all of which are lighter than anything fried and cheese-laden.

- Healthy salads include tossed, mixed green, fruit, or spinach. But watch the salad dressings. Try low-calorie, oil and vinegar, lemon juice, or order your favorite, just have it on the side.

- As an entree, you may want to opt for lean meats, poultry, or fish; prepared broiled, boiled, baked, grilled, charbroiled, roasted, steamed, or poached.

- If you're having a sandwich, go for turkey, chicken, lean meat, hamburger—grilled and plain—or tuna, but watch out for added mayonnaise.

- When ordering a la carte, select vegetables that are boiled, steamed, stir-fried, baked, or fresh without rich sauces or butter, and never fried.

- If you choose to have a potato, order it baked or boiled, without butter or sour cream on top.

- If you're having pasta, have any kind but without excess butter or cream sauces. Pasta is healthier for you if it comes with marinara sauce or any tomato-based sauce on the side.

Use less margarine when you saute, butter your vegetables, spread your bread, or top your casseroles. Skip it completely if you can. Try fat-free butter granules; they give you all the flavor and none of the fat.

- Hard rolls, breadsticks, tortilla chips, or crackers without added butter are better bread choices.

- And for dessert, try fresh fruit with raspberry or strawberry puree, or sorbet.

Dining Out Ethnic

Here are some tips for ordering when you dine at ethnic restaurants.

Good Choices in Chinese:

As an appetizer, try egg drop soup, wonton soup, hot and sour soup, or the inside ingredients of an egg roll. Don't eat that fried doughy exterior, though, it's loaded with fat.

For the entree, order stir-fried dishes rather than those that are breaded or fried and then served with sweet and sour sauces.

On the side, white rice or steamed vegetables are better choices than fried rice.

Eating Italian

Minestrone soup is your best bet in appetizers when you dine Italianne.

As an entree, consider thin-crust pizza instead of deluxe; pasta with marinara sauce instead of Alfredo or butter and cream-based sauces; baked or broiled veal or chicken instead of breaded Parmesan dishes.

Mexican Meals

Low-fat tortilla chips with salsa are a relatively low-fat appetizer. But, if you are also having a full meal, don't kill your appetite first. Ask the waiter to remove them if they are too tempting.

Cook vegetables only until they are crisp and tender to retain the vitamins. Microwave them with only one tablespoon of water for best results.

Good choices in Mexican entrees are dishes that include lots of vegetables, soft chicken tacos, or fajitas. Avoid dishes that contain loads of cheese; stay away from refried beans; meals made with lard are high-calorie and high-fat; and tamales are taboo.

A good Mexican side dish is beans and rice (if they're not cooked in lard). Try to limit your intake of guacamole, fried rice, and sour cream, which are often served on the side with Mexican entrees.

Dining on Quick Cuisine

Okay, we know fast foods, home-delivered meals, and take-out foods have become more and more popular with working women who want a quick bite for lunch or don't have time to prepare dinner. They are convenient, readily available, and usually less expensive than dine-in restaurants.

If you patronize the major fast-food chain restaurants, you can usually rely on consistent quality and taste, wherever you go, in large or small towns, and even in foreign countries. But is this "quick cuisine," as we call it, good for you? Well, you can work it into a healthy foodstyle if you learn to choose wisely and to balance fast fare with what you eat the rest of the day.

Get to know the nutritional values of your favorite fast-food items. The nutrient composition of similar foods can vary considerably among the chain restaurants because ingredients and cooking styles differ. Today the major chains offer nutrition information on their products. Ask for it at the restaurant. Once you know more about your favorites, you can incorporate them into your daily food plan.

Cut back on creamed and fried foods. Prepare your foods using healthier techniques such as baking, boiling, broiling, grilling, and steaming. Barbecuing, charcoaling, and shish-kebabing are also tasty choices.

Remember, many fast-food choices are high in fat, calories, sodium, and even sugar. Look for lower-fat options such as salad bars, low-fat salad dressings, broiled chicken fillets, and baked potatoes.

Here are some tips for "dining" a la "quick cuisine." Yes, it can be dining, if you take your time and enjoy the experience.

• You can have a 2-ounce hamburger on a bun with lettuce, tomato, dill pickles, and mustard for 300 calories or less. But, a 4-ounce hamburger with extras like sauce, cheese, or bacon, can range between 500 and 1000 calories.

- Most milkshakes have about 350 calories, but some have as many as 900 calories, depending on the size of the shake and the ingredients used by the restaurant. A glass of low-fat milk, on the other hand, has only 120 to 140 calories. Tea and coffee are calorie-free if you don't add cream or sugar. Most places have sugar substitutes available.

- Regular soft drinks offer little in the way of nutrition but can add 125 to 200 calories per 12-ounce serving. Most diet soft drinks contain less than 5 calories for a similar-sized serving.

There is no good or bad food. Variety, balance, and moderation are the keys to good nutrition.

- A small serving of French fries has about 200 calories. Fried onion rings contain about 275 calories per serving. A plain, small baked potato only adds about 120 calories to your daily intake. Large ones, though, can be as much as 250 calories.

- Catsup, pickles, mustard, and other condiments are high in sodium but relatively low in calories. Tartar sauce and mayonnaise are high in fat and calories. Using mustard instead of mayonnaise on your hamburger saves you about 150 calories.

- Pizza varies widely in calories depending on ingredients. The kind of crust makes a difference, too. A thick crust adds more calories. Sausage and pepperoni pizza is higher in calories, sodium, and fat than one topped with lean ground beef or vegetables. Two slices or one-fourth of a typical medium pizza has 300 to 400 calories.

- Fish and chicken are usually low in fat and calories, but breading and frying them convert them to not-so-healthy choices. A fried fish fillet sandwich has 400 to 500 calories; a sandwich made with a fried chicken fillet has even more. One tablespoon of tartar sauce adds 75 more calories; and one tablespoon of mayonnaise adds 100 calories. A 3-piece fried chicken dinner with mashed potatoes, gravy, coleslaw, roll, and butter can soar to 1000 calories, most of your day's needs in only one meal. An extra crispy dinner adds 100 calories more per piece of chicken.

Dining In, Dining Out, Dining Meatless 165

> *Use only small amounts of water when cooking vegetables. Vitamins and minerals may be lost if they seep into the water and are poured out. Steam vegetables in a glass bowl or microwave-safe dish, covered, until tender-crisp (about 5 to 6 minutes).*
>
> ～

- A large, plain baked potato has about 200 to 250 calories and is an excellent source of complex carbohydrates and fiber. But sour cream, bacon, cheese, and other tater-toppers can take that same healthy potato to an unhealthy 600 calories or more and it can be disastrous for your daily sodium levels. Instead, top that potato with vegetables or low fat cottage cheese.

- Cereal, English muffins, or bagels with jelly (not butter or margarine) make a much better breakfast selection than egg, sausage, and cheese sandwiches.

- Croissant sandwiches are delicious, but a croissant is considerably higher in fat and calories than a bun.

- A visit to the salad bar can be a healthy option. Lettuce and vegetables usually add up to around 60 to 100 calories. You can quickly destroy the lean-cuisine value of your healthy choice by adding a ladle of salad dressing, containing 200 to 250 calories, or by digging into the prepared salads made with mayonnaise.

- Mexican fast food is popular these days, but make your selections wisely. Tacos have 200 to 300 calories; enchiladas and burritos have 350 to 500. If you think you are being prudent by ordering a taco salad, think again. Most taco salads contain 600 to 1200 calories, depending on the ingredients and the amount of salad dressing you use. The average chalupa has 300 calories and a fajita about 275.

- Chinese fast food can be low in calories if you opt for stir-fried dishes. But beware of MSG (monosodium glutamate). Many Chinese restaurants use this high-in-sodium preservative in cooking. Ask to have it omitted. Soy sauce is also high in sodium, but many sit-down restaurants now have the low-sodium variety available.

Better Bites in Fast-Food Fare

Here's a summary to help you know how to make better choices when you go for fast foods.

Instead of:	Choose:	Save:
Pizza		
2 slices deluxe	2 slices cheese	122 calories
16-inch	16-inch	14 grams fat
498 cal/20 mg fat	376 cal/6 gm fat	
Hamburger		
double meat with cheese	single hamburger	440 calories
French fries	side salad w/light dressing	29 grams fat
870 cal/49 gm fat	430 cal/20 gm fat	
Steak		
6 oz. ribeye	5 oz. sirloin	319 calories
baked potato w/ margarine, sour cream	baked potato w/margarine	32 grams fat
toast	toast	
975 cal/58 gm fat	656 cal/26 gm fat	
Chicken		
extra crispy breast	rotisserie (no skin)	312 calories
mashed potatoes	baked beans or corn	23 grams fat
biscuit	coleslaw	
685 cal/39 gm fat	373 cal/16 gm fat	

Instead of:	Choose:	Save:
Mexican		
taco salad	chicken fajita	517 calories
pintos and cheese	432 cal/20 gm fat	42 grams fat
949 cal/62 gm fat		
Fish		
3-piece fried dinner	baked fish dinner	573 calories
w/ French fries, slaw	w/ vegetables, slaw	25 grams fat
hush puppies	387 cal/19 gm fat	
960 cal/44 gm fat		

Dining on the Road

Whether you are traveling on your job or just taking a family vacation, if you aren't careful about your dining choices, life on the road can destroy weeks or even months of careful eating. We all want to "pull out the stops" when we're out of town. It isn't unusual to find that you've consumed 4,000 to 5,000 calories in a day on the road, arriving home a bit thicker at the waistline and hips. This is especially so for conventioneers who seem to be on a gastronomic marathon, eating everything offered at each buffet meal.

Well, here's some advice for when you're on the road. First of all, don't eat three big meals a day. A light breakfast of fruit and cereal or a muffin and a lunch of salad with a roll and fruit will leave you plenty of calories to enjoy a lovely evening dinner.

Second, take your walking shoes and use them to burn up excess calories. Also, check out hotel health clubs. More and more exercise options are becoming available to travelers. Think you don't have time? Just get up 30 minutes earlier each morning and go work out.

Going on a cruise? You won't lose any weight on this vacation unless you are seasick most of the time! Cruise ships are known for fabulous food and you should plan to enjoy it. But that doesn't mean you should abandon your healthy foodstyle altogether. Work for balance. If you splurge at one meal, slack off a little at the next. Then, hit the deck and take a walk.

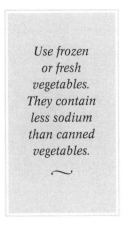

Use frozen or fresh vegetables. They contain less sodium than canned vegetables.

Many cruise ships have become more health conscious and now offer foods that are nutritious, tasty, and beautifully served. Some even offer spa cuisine and fitness programs because they recognize that it's not that easy for passengers to get as much exercise as they need to handle the variety and quantity of foods offered.

When you fly to your destination, take the time to order a special meal from the airline in advance. It costs nothing extra and can save you unwanted calories and fat. These arrangements must be made more than a day in advance, however, since these meals are specially prepared and it takes organization to get them onto the right flight in the right city at the right time.

Remember, however, flying can be fattening. Here's what we mean:

Calorie content of a typical hot airline meal = 1000

Calorie content of a typical snack meal = 300

Calorie content of 1-ounce package peanuts = 170

Calorie content of 1-ounce package pretzels = 100

Calorie content of 12-ounce cola drink = 155

Calorie content of 1 cocktail (minibottle, no mix) = 110

So, if you are flying from Akron, Ohio, to Minneapolis and you make a connection in Chicago, you probably consumed upwards of 1800 calories along the way. And when you leave the plane, you're likely to go to dinner! So be careful of calories in the air.

Pour browned ground beef in a colander to drain the fat off.

If you're traveling by car and the weather permits, take a picnic along with your favorite healthy foods. Take apples, grapes, or vegetables, and some water for drinking in the car. If you choose to stop and eat out, make your menu selections carefully. You won't be as active or need as many calories when you sit in a car all day. You'll feel a lot better and stay more alert if you don't overeat.

Of course, if you are on vacation, you deserve to enjoy dining at that special restaurant you've heard so much about. Splurging can be okay, but only if you are sensible and learn to balance your overall food intake.

On Being a Dinner Guest

Perhaps one of the most difficult times to stick with your new healthy foodstyle is when you are a guest for dinner at someone's home. It isn't easy to sit down at a friend's table and refuse foods you are offered. Nor is it polite. Unless you are on a specific diet, prescribed by a physician, consider this event a time to splurge. Eat, enjoy, and compliment the chef! But, before you go over for dinner, eat lightly. Remember, you can retain control by balancing your meals before and after the dinner-guest experience. Eat lean meals before and after the occasion.

If you have the option, take small servings, pass on seconds, and avoid the salt shaker and butter. These small moves will go unnoticed and will keep you on your road to good health.

Actually, today most of us are so aware of the relationship between what and how much we eat and our health that our hosts also are taking this into account. If you run into a difficult situation, however, just enjoy yourself. There's no need to feel guilty or out of control. After all, as Scarlett O'Hara said, "Tomorrow is another day."

"My Compliments to the Cook"

Most of this book is about those times when you cook at home and how to manage a healthy foodstyle and a hectic lifestyle. Now we want to give you some tips for those times when you invite your friends into your home to "dine" with you. After all, sharing your home and your hospitality with others is one of the best compliments you can give to your friends.

Everyone pretty much recognizes that healthy dining is here to stay. Eating lighter, more nutritious fare is more than just a trend, far more than a fad, it is why we call it "foodstyle." It is part of the overall healthy lifestyles we all are working to adopt. Cooking light, with style, can make you everyone's favorite hostess.

Plan the meal so that you emphasize the leisurely aspect of dining. Entertaining can be informal but still comfortably elegant. Try involving your guests in the preparations and in the serving. Experiment with recipes from the new low-fat cookbooks available at bookstores or try the ideas we've included here.

Components in strawberries may protect against certain types of cancer. Strawberries are low in calories and high in fiber and vitamin C.

You can serve "theme" dinners or try ethnic cooking at home. You can even get your friends organized for progressive dinners where you have appetizers at one home, entrees at another, and dessert at yet another. Make your at-home dinner parties festive and fun.

Dining Meatless

The vegetarian foodstyle, once uncommon, has become a very popular diet option for many. Whether you decide to become a vegan for religious or ethnic reasons, to avoid harming animals, or for health reasons, meatless diets, followed appropriately, can be a healthy choice when compared to the typically high-in-fat, low-in-fiber diet of most Americans.

Diets consisting of fruits, vegetables, whole grains, and dairy products can provide enough protein and all the essential nutrients we need. Non-vegetarian diets containing too many meat products can contain excess fat, cholesterol, no fiber, and have been linked to various forms of cancer, heart disease, diverticulosis, obesity, and even osteoporosis.

But, don't think that choosing a vegetarian foodstyle will put you on the path to good health automatically. Without making careful food selections, vegetarian diets can be low in calcium, iron, zinc, and vitamins A, D, and B12. You can also eat too much fat if you include lots of cheese, whole milk and dairy products, cream, margarine, and eggs, all of which can cause dietary concern. Only eating pasta with red sauce or bagels at meals will not give you the protein and iron you need each day.

Use a paper towel, cold lettuce leaf, or spoon to skim fat off soups, stews, sauces, and broths. You'll save more than 125 calories for each tablespoon of fat you remove.

You should select low-fat products such as low-fat milk, yogurt, and low- or nonfat dairy products, and add them to a diet of whole grain breads, cereals, pasta, crackers, legumes, dried beans and peas, and fruits and vegetables. Refer to the Food Guide Pyramid for the appropriate number of daily servings and portion sizes.

If you opt for the vegetarian foodstyle, your dietary possibilities are virtually limitless. But, be smart. Learn more about basic nutrition and plan your meals carefully. Read literature and cookbooks for ideas. Enjoy your food at the same time as you improve your diet and health.

Remember, whether you're dining out at a four-star restaurant, a fast-food chain, or a friend's home, you don't have to give up all the foods you like. Enjoy yourself, make balance your basic philosophy of food, and live vibrant, young, and healthy ever after.

9 Medical Fact or Fiction?

Who to Believe When it Comes to Your Health

Did you know that health fraud and quackery are a $25 billion industry? And who do you think is most often the victim of health fraud? You guessed it: women. Every one of us is vulnerable when it comes to wanting a quick fix for our health challenges, aches and pains, or weight problems. But, the bad news is, there just aren't any fast fixes for most health problems. They didn't appear overnight and they can't be fixed overnight.

To complicate matters, misinformation about nutrition seems to be everywhere. We read it in magazines, see ads about it on TV, and find our mailboxes jammed with it. People claiming to be scientists or food experts even have their own TV shows. Or you find cable channels filled with so-called "infomercials" that are disguised as TV shows.

Many women turn to alternative physicians, some of whom may not really be physicians. Others head for health-food stores, looking for a vitamin or mineral cure-all for whatever is bothering them at the time.

Everyone suffers from minor aches and pains sometime. We are all under stress, and stress takes its toll on the human body. And, the process of aging is itself relentless, creeping up on us all. But, none of these constitutes illness, and beware of anyone who claims that these natural processes make you somehow mysteriously "ill."

Nutrition counselors cannot be expected to guarantee you that you will be spared from illnesses such as cancer or stroke. If you find one who does, think twice about going back. Nutritionists can't cure illness, but dietary intervention in the case of diabetes or high blood pressure may lessen the severity and progression of the disease.

If a counselor uses an emotional appeal, making you feel frightened or depressed, find someone who offers facts instead. Be wary of nutritionists who belittle the medical community, the Food and Drug Administration, or other governmental agencies. Most professionals have a great deal of respect for colleagues. And, beware the counselor who suggests "cytotoxic blood testing," "hair analysis," large doses of nutritional supplements, or "cleansing" with enemas.

Be a Health-Fraud Sleuth

Here's a list of tips from the Food and Drug Administration (FDA) and the Council of Better Business Bureaus that can help you separate fact from fiction when it comes to health claims.

- Be wary if a product's label or advertising promises immediate, effortless, or guaranteed results.

- Be wary of testimonials in ads or on labels from satisfied users. They can rarely be confirmed.

- Don't be taken in by "money-back" guarantees. A guarantee is only as good as the company that backs it.

- Be wary of promises of complete relief from pain.

- Don't be taken in by promises that any product offers a "cure."

- Watch out for claims that a treatment or product has been approved by the FDA. Federal law does not permit mention of the FDA in any way that suggests marketing approval for any drug or medical device.

- Don't give too much importance to the term "natural" to describe ingredients or preparations. The definition of "natural" is elusive, and the word is often abused.

- Look out for other misleading words such as amazing, secret, miracle, special, vanish, painless, discovery, breakthrough, exclusive, instant, immediate, quick, or fast.

- If the product sounds too good to be true, it probably is.

Use reduced-sodium products such as light soy sauce, low-sodium Worcestershire sauce, and reduced-sodium soups. One teaspoon of regular Worcestershire sauce has about 70 milligrams of sodium, while the low-sodium variety has only 20 milligrams.

How to Protect Yourself

Looking to increase your intake of calcium? Try these high calcium foods: milk, yogurt, cheese, dark green leafy vegetables, broccoli, and salmon.

~

The American Dietetic Association suggests that your best defense against health fraud is becoming an informed health-care consumer. Nutrition is an ever-changing science; what we know today may change in the future as we learn more. When you read or hear of some new discovery in nutrition, check it out. Often claims are made based on limited preliminary speculation about a nutrient or a food. While great discoveries make great headlines, be alert to whether the claim is actually backed by significant research or just a theory wanting research.

The most accurate information and guidance should come to you from your physician or a registered dietitian. Registered dietitians (R.D.) are recognized in the medical community as legitimate providers of nutrition health care. They will answer openly when you ask about their credentials, schooling, years of experience in nutrition counseling, and most recent training. They will give you realistic advice and usable information, with no mysteries and no claims of miracles.

Lose Weight Overnight! and Other Schemes

In the search for longevity, health, and vitality, many women in particular have become susceptible to buying into false claims of quick weight loss. In fact, weight loss has become a multi-billion dollar business in the U.S. It is practically the national pastime.

About half of all households in America include someone on a diet. Yet only 5 to 10 percent of the people who lose weight on one fad diet or another actually keep that weight off for more than five years. This should tell us something about any diet that promises easy, fast weight loss.

If there is one nutrition topic that is shrouded in mystery, it is how to lose weight. Every week there is some new approach to slimming down: the Three-Day diet, the Speed-Up-Your-Metabolism diet, the Burn-Up-Fat-by-Eating-Acid-Foods-like-Grapefruit diet, and on and on.

How do you recognize a fad diet? Well, if any diet makes a spectacular promise such as "eat all you want," "spot reduce," "prevent aging," or melt away fat," you can be sure the program has no scientific basis. Be wary of diets that offer quick, effortless weight loss without reducing calories and increasing exercise. Steer clear of diets based on the use of pills, "secret" formula powders, or the use or exclusion of various food groups. And, if any diet says you shouldn't stay on it for any extended period, it's not a good choice for your long-term health.

Low-calorie fad diets promise "painless" solutions to persistent problems. Sometimes these diets work at first because they put the dieter on such a strict food regimen. Most diets work initially, but the key to long-term success is to make changes in your eating behavior and your lifestyle.

Very low-calorie diets provide less than 800 calories daily. These diets are designed for extreme cases of obesity and should be used only under strict medical supervision. You will certainly lose weight on such a limited program, but you can do serious damage to your body if you attempt this without medical support.

Very low-calorie diets can result in weight loss, but what kind of weight are you losing? Will it stay off? Be sure any diet you consider has the following essential components:

- medical supervision
- nutrition education
- behavior modification
- lifestyle education

> *Make nutritious snacks a part of your foodstyle: fruits, juices, bagels, rice cakes, low-fat yogurt, raw vegetables, pretzels, and popcorn.*

Some of the most popular weight-loss schemes around today are named after famous people, places, and gimmicks. These diets usually focus on a few foods or food combinations. They are often nutritionally deficient and, because of this, they tend to promote binge eating and dietary imbalance.

There are also commercial franchise businesses that charge weekly fees for dietary counseling and support. Some of these practice sound nutritional principles; some do not. Sometimes these businesses supply you with food for the program; sometimes they do not. Some provide supplements, liquid "diet food," or herbal capsules. Be wary of the latter.

The costs of these programs are often hidden, which means the price per pound lost can be very high. Don't use these programs just for the weight loss they offer, make a profit on your investment: learn as much as you can about nutrition and exercise. Take advantage of every opportunity to learn how to keep the weight off forever. Watch to see if your behaviors are changing for the better and for good. Be alert to opportunities to develop your life-long foodstyle.

You can judge whether you are getting your money's worth if:

1. you experience a steady weight loss of one to two pounds a week and that weight lost is really fat, not muscle or water loss;
2. your program includes a nutritionally balanced, but calorie-reduced, meal plan with no fewer than 1,200 calories and foods from all the major food groups on the Food Guide Pyramid;
3. you receive encouragement to increase your physical activity level to reasonable levels;

4. you get all the help you need in assessing your eating habits and identifying problem areas, and you get the education and support you need to promote positive changes in your eating habits.

The secret to vibrant, young, and healthy living that lasts a long time is keeping your eye on the big picture. Think of your health, not just your weight. In your personal diet or foodstyle, it's the overall intake of nutrients over several days that counts. It's not just for today; it's not just for tomorrow. It's for the rest of your life.

Have a bird hunter in the family? Wild duck, pheasant, quail, and dove are very low in fat.

Foods to Stay Vibrant, Young & Healthy

10 Special Health Concerns

N o two women are exactly alike, and as we age, our differences, physically, increase. Each of us has a different set of experiences, different lifestyle, and different likes and dislikes, in addition. Thus we are each unique. And that holds true for our nutritional needs, too, although we all need the same basic nutrients to survive. Our individual requirements for optimum health, however, can be as unique as we are. Consequently we each have our own special health concerns. Understanding nutrition and its relationship to these concerns can help us manage whatever those special needs might be.

Here's a rundown of some common health conditions women confront.

Anemia

Women are prime candidates for anemia, a condition where there is a deficiency of hemoglobin (the red cells) in the blood to carry oxygen around the body. In order to form red cells, we need the mineral iron and the water-soluble vitamins folic acid and vitamin B12.

Why are women at particular risk for anemia?

There are a number of reasons, including:

- Menstruation: Blood loss on a monthly basis may lead to iron deficiency.

- Pregnancy: The increase in blood volume (3 pints or more of blood) with pregnancy increases the need for iron to supply red blood cells. Folic acid demand is greater for the development of the baby.

- New Mothers: Following delivery of the baby, an increased iron supply is needed to replenish the mother's iron stores.

- Dietary Deficiency: Women tend to have less iron in their diets because fewer total calories are consumed, in general, to maintain a stable weight. Many women complicate this deficiency by going on calorie-restrictive diets to lose weight.

What are the symptoms of anemia?

If you are anemic, you will experience some, if not all, of the following:

- Lack of energy;
- Tiredness or constant fatigue;
- Paleness of the skin;
- Shortness of breath on exertion;
- Vitamin B12 deficiency

How much iron do you need?

The Recommended Dietary Allowance for iron in women is:

Up to age 50—15 milligrams

Age 51 plus—10 milligrams

During pregnancy—30 milligrams

During lactation—15 milligrams

If you suspect that you may be anemic, you should see your physician for a blood test to measure your hemoglobin and/or hematocrit level.

How can I treat anemia?

Obviously, the best treatment for anemia is prevention, and that includes eating iron-rich foods regularly during your menstrual years. So, treatment may include the addition of iron-rich foods to your diet, with possible use of an iron supplement. These foods include dark green, leafy vegetables, fish, red meat, liver, enriched cereals and whole grains, and dried fruits.

The benefits of foods high in iron are increased by adding foods rich in vitamin C at the same meal. Vitamin C is known to increase the absorption of iron into the bloodstream. Vitamin C-rich foods are orange juice, citrus fruits, broccoli, green peppers, and tomatoes, among others.

The following is a sample daily menu plan rich in iron.

Pumping Iron

Food	Serving Size	Iron (mg)	Calories	Fat (gm)
Breakfast				
Cream of wheat	1 cup	11	140	<1
raisins	1 Tbsp.	0.2	41	<1
low-fat milk	1 cup	0.1	102	5
margarine	1 tsp.	0	34	4
Lunch				
salad of—				
romaine lettuce	1 cup	0.6	9	<1
spinach	1 cup	1.5	12	<1
kidney beans	1/4 cup	0.8	52	<1
chick-peas	1/4 cup	1	67	1
green peas	1/4 cup	0.3	31	—
tomato	1/2	0.3	13	—
Ranch dressing	2 Tbsp.	0.1	110	11
crackers	4	0.5	50	3

Pumping Iron, continued

Food	Serving Size	Iron (mg)	Calories	Fat (gm)
Dinner				
roast beef	3 oz.	2.2	204	14
lima beans	1/2 cup	1.76	94	<1
baked potato with skin on	1 medium	2.75	220	<1
margarine	1 tsp.	0	34	4
Snacks				
popcorn made in an air popper	1 cup	0.2	30	<1
low-fat yogurt	1/2 cup	0.1	110	1
plums	3 small	0.9	47	<1
Totals		*26 gm*	*1400 calories*	*43 gm*

Arthritis

So far, researchers have found no specific food or diet that will cure arthritis, but the basic principles of good nutrition and proper weight maintenance are essential to lighten the burden on inflamed arthritic joints.

Arthritis has been known to us since antiquity. It is not just a single disease, but many. Real cures are rare, but we have learned that the condition can be controlled. Many women with arthritis have learned to bear some discomfort and still lead normal lives. Stages of remission are common with arthritis, and can make you think you have been cured. As with other health conditions, there is always some irresponsible marketeer ready to sell you some "cure." But don't be misled, people with arthritis pay about $400 million each year on fraudulent cures, treatments, and devices.

Misinformation related to diet and arthritis makes reference to "miracle foods," including sea water, "immune" milk, honey and apple cider combinations, alfalfa tablets, and large doses of vitamin preparations. In truth, there is no valid scientific evidence linking any food or supplement with control or cure of arthritis. The one exception to this is the relationship between food and obesity, malnourishment, or fluid retention.

Obesity complicates osteoarthritis, which is an enlargement or stiffening of the joints that comes with aging. Extra weight causes a burden on arthritic joints, thus increasing inflammation and pain. A weight-reduction diet designed by a registered dietitian can help control obesity and ensure that the essential nutrients are provided. Women with osteoarthritis also tend to have less calcium in their bones and often suffer from a mild form of anemia, as well. A diet rich in calcium from low-fat milk and dairy products and high in iron from lean meat and other iron sources can help alleviate both calcium deficiencies and anemia.

Rheumatoid arthritis, a chronic and progressive inflammatory tissue disorder, may cause weight loss and undernourishment. This condition is helped with an increase in protein-rich foods like such as cheese, meat, fish, and dried beans. High-calorie foods are often recommended until weight is back to normal.

If you are managing arthritis of any kind, your physician is your best source of information. Your physician will help you decide whether you need a specific food or vitamin supplements. Your basic guideline should be to eat wisely and maintain a desirable body weight. Your food-style management will help you meet the physical demands arthritis presents and, even with arthritis, you can feel vibrant, young, and healthy.

Cancer

Today we are bombarded with information about what to eat or not eat to prevent cancer. Recent headlines causing public concern call attention to possible relationships between fiber and cancer, pesticides and cancer, antioxidants and cancer, and general diet and cancer.

You need to be very careful to separate what is scientific fact from unfounded theory. When diet and cancer research contains suppositions ("maybes" and "mights"), be suspicious. Always evaluate any data or source to verify its validity. The National Council Against Health Fraud, Inc., P.O. Box 1276, Loma Linda, California 92345, is a good source when you have questions, as are county and state consumer protection offices. Only one thing is really certain: we don't yet know the cause of many forms of cancer.

We do know, however, that the word "cancer" really describes a group of over 200 different dis-

Olive oil (a good fat) helps prevent coronary artery disease by maintaining HDL levels (the good cholesterol). Because olive oil is still a fat, limit yourself to 1 or 2 teaspoons a day.

eases. Most experts today agree that there is a link between smoking and lung cancer. And most are certain that over-exposure to sunlight causes skin cancer. But no specific food is known to cause or cure any form of cancer. Today, however, there is some evidence that certain components of the diet may aid in cancer prevention. The American Cancer Society (ACS) and other scientists have issued some nutrition guidelines in this area.

- The ACS reports that obesity is associated with a greater risk of cancer of the uterus, gall bladder, kidney, stomach, prostate, colon, and breast. Although this connection cannot be attributed solely to dietary fat, the ACS does endorse limiting fat to 30 percent of total daily calories.

- A diet high in fiber may help reduce the risk of colon cancer, although this connection remains somewhat controversial. It is likely, however, that if you eat a diet high in fiber—fruits, vegetables, and grains—you probably will be eating less fat, which may also reduce colon cancer risk.

- The ACS also recommends eating foods rich in vitamins A and C. Some studies have indicated that foods rich in beta carotene, which is converted to vitamin A in the liver, lower the risk of cancer of the larynx, esophagus, and lungs. People who consume foods rich in vitamin C or ascorbic acid are less likely to get cancer of the stomach and esophagus, but it is still uncertain whether vitamin C itself, or other constituents of foods containing vitamin C, have the protective effect.

- Current interest has focused on antioxidants, including beta carotene, vitamin C, vitamin E, and the mineral selenium, and their role in preventing heart disease and cancer, as well as slowing down the aging process itself. Antioxidants neutralize "free radicals" present in the body. Free radicals are unstable forms of oxygen molecules that can combine randomly with components of healthy cells, interfering with normal cell growth and activity.

It is this interference that is thought to cause some forms of cancer and premature aging of body cells.

Studies show that groups of people eating foods high in antioxidants, such as sweet potatoes, spinach, broccoli, kale, cantaloupe, strawberries, kiwi fruit, and citrus fruits tend to have lower rates of cancer and heart disease. While the experts are not convinced that taking antioxidants in pill or capsule form is effective, many recommend a meal plan abundant in foods rich in antioxidants.

Food Sources of Antioxidants

Vegetables/Fruit—

Sweet potatoes, broccoli, kale, spinach, brussels sprouts, carrots, red cabbage, squash, cantaloupe, strawberries, kiwifruit, citrus fruit, apricots, peaches, and watermelon

Breads/Cereals—

Whole grain breads and cereals, pumpernickel, corn bread, muffins, crackers, oats, barley, and brown rice

Fish/Seafood—

Cod, halibut, lobster, shrimp, salmon, scallops, swordfish, and tuna

- A number of studies have demonstrated that cruciferous vegetables—such as cabbage, broccoli, brussels sprouts, and cauliflower—reduce the risk of gastrointestinal and respiratory tract cancer. It is not yet clear exactly what in these foods has the protective effect.

- It has also been suggested that sulfur-containing substances, called sulfides, in garlic and onions, may inhibit cancer. The American Institute for Cancer Research is currently funding research to explore this potential link.

- Foods that are smoked, such as ham and some varieties of sausage, fish, and turkey, are considered possible players in an increased risk of cancer. Tars that arise from wood or charcoal fires used to smoke these foods may contain carcinogens. This warning may apply to some bar-becuing, too, but there probably is no great danger in eating char-broiled foods occasionally.

- Nitrate-cured foods also have been cited as possible links to cancer. Nitrate is traditionally used to preserve meat and improve its color and flavor. After a great deal of research, the U.S. Department of Agriculture and the American meat industry have lowered the amount of nitrate used as a preservative. Both are searching for improved methods to guarantee a safe food supply. Other chemicals added to food to improve color and flavor and prevent spoilage are also under scrutiny. So far there's not enough evidence to recommend avoiding them.

- Use of artificial sweeteners has been addressed by the American Cancer Society, but so far no specific recommendations have been made. Currently, all artificial sweetners on the market are listed on the FDA's GRAS (generally recognized as safe) list. Studies failed to prove that saccharin use caused cancer in humans, but bladder tumors were found in rats who were given huge doses.

- There is some evidence that phytochemicals (non-nutrient com-pounds found in food) may help protect against heart disease, some types of cancer, and complications associated with diabetes. Phytochemicals appear in all plant foods. It's best to get them through varied food choices—rather than through a supplemental form. A well-rounded diet will provide a wide variety of nutrients and non-nutrients necessary for health and well-being.

It is believed that most cancers develop either in response to two or more different causes or because specific individuals are particularly sus-ceptible to specific forms of it, either through genetic predisposition or exposure to toxins. Planning your diet around suggested guidelines may help prevent cancer, but diet itself will rarely be solely responsible for prevention. You can control the odds when you manage your foodstyle, so why not hedge your bets? Eat smart.

Food Sources of Phytochemicals

Vegetables/Fruit—

Apples, apricots, berries, cantaloupe, citrus fruits, grapes; bok choy, broccoli, brussels sprouts, cabbage, carrots, cauliflower, celery, collards, cucumber, eggplant, garlic, kale, onions, parsnips, peppers, tomatoes, turnips

Breads/Cereals—

Whole wheat bread, barley, brown rice, oats

Protein Rich Foods—

Black beans, kidney beans, pinto beans, soybeans, tofu

Breast Cancer

Breast cancer, the most frequently diagnosed cancer in women, strikes about 182,000 women each year in the U.S. Of those, it kills 46,000. One in eight women will develop breast cancer. Here are some facts:

- The incidence of breast cancer has increased 3 percent per year since 1960. Some increase is believed due to improved screening methods which lead to earlier and more accurate diagnoses.

- The five-year survival rate has increased from 78 percent in the 1940s to 91 percent today. If the cancer has not spread, the survival rate is 100 percent.

- Mammograms (low-dose breast X-rays) are considered a valuable diagnostic tool, yet they are estimated to miss 15 to 20 percent of those with breast cancer. Most experts recommend a three-step approach to early diagnosis and subsequent prevention:

1. Clinical exams by a physician during regular health checkups;
2. Mammograms as recommended—baseline mammogram between ages 35 and 39; mammograms every 1 to 2 years for ages 40 to 49; and every year after age 50;
3. Regular self-breast examination performed once a month at the same time each month.

Age, early onset of menstrual periods, late age of first pregnancy, late menopause, family history, and obesity are known risk factors, but they account for only 40 to 50 percent of all breast cancers. The cause of the other 50 to 60 percent remains a mystery.

Does fat cause breast cancer? Does nutrition play some role?

There is probably no research area more controversial than the possible link between breast cancer and nutrition, particularly between breast cancer and dietary fat intake. But study results are still conflicting. Nothing to date is conclusive. Diet may well make a difference between promotion of, or prevention of, breast cancer. We simply don't know. Until further research provides better understanding, health experts recommend that all women eat a diet low in fat especially saturated fat (that means less than 30 percent total fat for women at low risk; less than 20 percent for women at high risk), high in fiber, and high in fruits and vegetables. In addition, alcohol should be consumed only in moderate amounts (less than two drinks a day), and weight kept in a healthy range. These good eating habits will help women beat the odds against breast cancer and heart disease.

Fresh, raw vegetables are a "fast food" requiring little or no preparation (except washing).

~

Chronic Fatigue Syndrome

Little research has been done about chronic fatigue syndrome (CFS), a debilitating condition of increasing fatigue and tiredness. Diet and nutritional status have not yet been linked to CFS as a proven treatment or cure. Nor are megavitamins, mineral supplements, or diets that eliminate certain foods the way to go, despite the fact that you may see testimonials, anecdotal evidence, and self-help books claiming the contrary. Until conclusive research tells us otherwise, your best bet is to try to make the healthiest food choices you can.

Diabetes

The American Diabetes Association reports that while 85 percent of the population has been tested for high blood pressure in the last three years, less than half have been tested for diabetes. They also note that 13 million Americans have diabetes, yet only 6.5 million cases have been diagnosed.

Diabetes is a disease of inadequate blood glucose (sugar) regulation, usually caused by insufficient or relatively ineffective insulin, a hormone produced in the pancreas.

Type I Diabetes

There are two forms of diabetes. The first, known as Type I diabetes, or insulin-dependent diabetes mellitus (IDDM), is less common, accounting for only 5 to 10 percent of all cases. This form of diabetes is sometimes called juvenile diabetes. The pancreas in IDDM, for some unknown reason, becomes unable to make insulin. After each meal, blood sugar rises and remains high while the body's cells are simultaneously starved for glucose (energy). The function of insulin is to move blood sugar into the body's cells. Insulin must be injected because stomach acid digests oral insulin before it can reach the bloodstream.

Type I diabetes usually is diagnosed in people under the age of 30 who are lean and who often have just experienced a rapid weight loss accompanied by symptoms of excessive thirst, excessive urination, hunger, and blurred vision.

Type I diabetes affects men and women alike. Treatment requires daily insulin injections (often 2 to 4 times) to assist the cells in taking in the blood sugar necessary, dietary management, and scheduled exercise. It is not unusual for people with diabetes to have sudden drops in blood sugar. This occurrence, known as hypoglycemia, requires quick treatment with food, especially a fast-acting carboydrate such as juice or candy.

Recent research has brought new understanding and hope to those with diabetes. The Diabetes Control and Complications Trial (DCCT), sponsored by the National Institutes of Health, was designed to answer one pressing question: Does tight control of blood sugar levels slow or prevent complications associated with diabetes? The answer is yes!

Brown rice, couscous, and whole wheat pasta are healthy substitutes for white rice and pasta. To get the benefit of whole grains, replace white flour with whole wheat or a mixture of whole wheat and white when you bake.

The 10-year study ended in 1993 and involved more than 1400 patients with results so clear cut that the study was stopped ahead of schedule. The findings were nothing short of spectacular. There was a 70-percent reduction in retinopathy (a condition of the eyes that can lead to blindness), a 50-percent reduction in nephropathy (kidney disease), and a 60-percent reduction in neuropathy (nerve disease) with tight control of blood sugar levels.

Thus, the study proved that tight control of blood sugar prevents or delays complications of Type I diabetes, some of the leading causes of death or disability for people with Type I diabetes. The study further recommended intensive therapy for most patients. With Type I diabetes, intensive therapy includes multiple daily injections of insulin or the use of an insulin pump, and frequent self blood glucose monitoring.

Type II Diabetes

The second type of diabetes, the most common, accounts for 90 percent of all cases. This is known as Type II or noninsulin-dependent diabetes mellitus. It is characterized by insulin impairment and insulin resistance. Insulin, produced in the pancreas, is usually present in the bloodstream in Type II diabetes, but it moves sugar for energy to the cells too slowly. Many people with Type II diabetes take insulin injections or insulin stimulating pills to supplement their own body supply.

Type II diabetes appears later in life (usually in those over 40) and is more likely to develop in overweight people (80 percent of all cases). There is usually a family history of diabetes. Obesity in this case is complicated by overeating. Because the cells are not getting the glucose they need for energy, people with Type II diabetes tend to eat more, trying desperately to get some energy. The overeating causes weight gain, causing the body to need even more energy, while the cells continue to resist the inadequate insulin available. Thus a vicious cycle is begun. Fat cells become larger and more demanding and even more insulin resistant, so the person often eats more and gains more weight.

The treatment for Type II diabetes is weight loss, even a moderate weight loss of 10 to 20 pounds, combined with increased physical activity. Sadly, for many women in particular, these two things are very hard to do. Changing a lifestyle takes education and effort. But 25 percent of those people with Type II diabetes can control their blood sugar levels with calorie control, proper spacing of meals, and regular exercise.

Some people may not be able to control their diabetes this easily and may need additional treatment, such as oral medications or daily doses of insulin. But the first step, and cornerstone of treatment, is meal planning and regular exercise.

Other Types of Diabetes

Gestational diabetes, the occurrence of diabetes during pregnancy, is usually treated with a meal plan, and sometimes with supplemental insulin. It is found in 2 to 5 percent of all pregnancies and usually disappears after delivery. Some women with gestational diabetes eventually develop Type II diabetes later in life, particularly if they become overweight and do not exercise.

Impaired glucose tolerance, sometimes called borderline diabetes, occurs when blood sugar levels rise above the normal range. About 25 percent of people with impaired glucose tolerance eventually develop Type II diabetes.

Frequent or ongoing hypoglycemia, or low blood sugar, may also be a precursor to Type II diabetes. This condition should always be investigated because it may be an indicator of other medical problems. A small percentage of diabetes cases are caused by other medical conditions such as pancreatitis, hormonal disturbances, or excessive use of steroids, among others.

Managing Diabetes

All in all, proper nutrition and consistent eating patterns is the answer to blood sugar control. But, if you have diabetes, you already know that good control requires training and reshaping of lifelong eating habits. Because of the complications diabetes may cause later in life, however, getting in control is worth it.

Diabetes not only affects the metabolism of carbohydrates, protein, and fat, but also the structure of the blood vessels and nerves in the body. It can lead to impaired circulation, impaired vision, and a loss of sensation in the arms and legs. When diabetes is poorly managed, infection is frequent, since bacteria thrive on sugar-rich blood. Often limbs with less feeling become havens for infection.

Strokes and heart attacks are likely when circulation is impaired. In fact, women with diabetes are at far greater risk of heart disease than men with diabetes. Women with diabetes are 150 percent more at risk than men for heart attack. Risk of sudden death from heart attack is 300 percent higher for women with diabetes, and women with diabetes have four times the risk of death from heart disease than men with diabetes.

What can be done to reduce these risks?

As we've said, nutrition and exercise, combined with medications as required, is the best way to normalize blood sugar levels and reduce, delay, or avoid the serious complications of diabetes. A healthy meal plan and exercise schedule tailored to each individual woman with diabetes by a registered dietitian and diabetes educator is in order. Frequent blood glucose monitoring may also be required.

New nutrition guidelines for diabetes have recently been developed that promote flexible meal plans. For a long time, nutrition experts and researchers thought simple sugars such as candy, pop, and other sweets were off limits to people with diabetes. These foods were believed to raise blood sugar too quickly. New research, however, proved that simple sugars do not raise blood sugar any quicker than starches. In fact, all carbohydrates (sugars and starches) are digested and in the bloodstream within 1 to 1 1/2 hours. So, small portions of simple sugars can be worked into a diabetes meal plan.

Another new surprising recommendation is, "There is no one diet for diabetes." General guidelines for healthy eating using the Food Guide Pyramid are the building blocks of a diabetes meal plan to manage blood sugar, blood fats, and blood pressure and to reach a reasonable weight. Tailoring a meal plan around individual calorie and nutrient needs as well as schedule and lifestyle has replaced the rigid and sometimes impractical preprinted diet sheets.

Just as no one diabetes diet exists, there is no one approach to meal planning and increasing physical activity. Registered dietitians and certified diabetes educators can help people with diabetes develop a plan to fit their needs and one that can be followed for a long time. For more information on how to find a diabetes educator, call the American Association of Diabetes Educators at (800) 338-3633.

Meal Planning for Successful Diabetes Management

- Have the best blood glucose readings possible

	Normal	**Acceptable**
Fasting (before breakfast)	80-120 mg/dL	less than 140
2 hrs. after meals	less than 140	less than 180
Hemoglobin A1c test (6-8 week average)	less than 6%	less than 7.5

- Reach your best activity level to help control blood sugar and take advantage of other important health benefits.
- Eat moderate portions.
- Strive for consistency, in meal times and in calorie intake from day to day.
- Eat foods from all of the food groups of the Food Guide Pyramid. Try new foods and go for variety.

Gastrointestinal Disorders

One common gastrointestinal disorder, diverticulosis, is characterized by the formation of pockets along weakened areas of the large intestinal wall. These pockets may resemble blowout spots in a tire and can become infected with the accumulation of food particles.

Diverticulosis tends to be common among those who habitually consume low-fiber diets. Consequently, a diet high in fiber is often the treatment for this condition. High-fiber foods increase the volume and weight of materials reaching these pockets and help keep them free from food particles.

Substances in tofu and soy products have been known to help reduce the incidence of cancer and reduce symptoms that accompany menopause.

High-fiber foods also can be useful in treating constipation. As we get older, our lives become more stressful, the tone of the intestinal smooth muscles diminishes, and the activity of the intestinal tract lessens. The resulting constipation is not only uncomfortable, but also potentially serious. Constipation also can be caused by a low-fiber diet as well as inadequate exercise and intake of fluids.

However, there is a down side to a sudden increase of high-fiber foods in the diet. You may feel stuffed or bloated. If you eat excessive amounts of fiber without giving your body a chance to adjust, your colon may have difficulty adapting to the rapid change. It's best to increase fiber gradually to save yourself from the discomforts of gas, cramps, and perhaps diarrhea. Select your fiber from a variety of food sources and eat it throughout the day. For best results, remember to drink 6 to 8 glasses of water daily. Fiber supplements may also be recommended by your doctor.

Heart Disease

The United States has one of the highest death rates from cardiovascular disease in the world. Heart attacks and strokes are the number one killers of American women. After age 50, nearly 500,000 women in the U.S. die of cardiovascular disease annually. Compare that with the deaths of 222,000 women from all forms of cancer.

Women who fall victim to heart attacks are twice as likely to die within two weeks following the attack than their male counterparts. Additionally, women who survive are at a greater risk than men to have a second heart attack. So, overall, heart disease affects men and women equally. The myth that heart disease affects men, not women, stems from the fact that few women develop severe heart disease before menopause. Heart disease in women has simply not received as much public attention.

Being a woman has some small advantage, at least in terms of heart health, but only early on in life. That is, being a woman delays, but does not prevent, heart disease. The incidence of heart attacks and coronary artery disease is much more common in middle-aged and older men than in premenopausal women. Women under 45 years of age suffer only about 3,000 heart attacks yearly, nationwide. But the risk increases with age. Only one in nine women between 45 and 64 develop heart disease, but the rate increases to an alarming one in three after the age of 65— almost equal to the incidence of heart disease in men of the same age.

The explanation? It has been noted that a woman's natural estrogen may protect her against heart problems prior to menopause. Hormone replacement therapy may thus prolong this protection. The exact mechanisms affording this protection remain unknown, but learning more about heart disease and how to prevent it using a healthful foodstyle is part of vibrant, young, and healthy living.

Coronary heart disease is a condition of the heart and blood vessels in which the coronary arteries become clogged with fatty, fibrous, cholesterol-laden deposits. The chief cause of coronary heart disease is atherosclerosis, which occurs when build-up of deposits cause the artery walls to thicken and the channel of the vessels to narrow. The flow of oxygen-rich blood through the arteries is decreased, resulting in inadequate blood supply to the heart. Sometimes this condition causes chest pain known as angina pectoris, which radiates to the left shoulder or arm during physical exertion. Angina pectoris is an early indicator of coronary heart disease but it usually does not occur until the passageway of the coronary artery is reduced by at least 50 percent.

What are the risks for women? Which are most important?

A key element in coronary health is cholesterol, the fat-like substance found in foods of animal origin. Since it is fat-like, cholesterol does not mix well with water and is transported in the bloodstream in little packages called lipoproteins. Lipoproteins are composed of various amounts of cholesterol, triglycerides, and other proteins. The names of two lipoproteins are now fairly common words: low-density lipoproteins (LDL) and high-density lipoproteins (HDL).

Low-density lipoproteins seem to attract cholesterol. Even though cholesterol has the same characteristics wherever it is found, the cholesterol found in LDL tends to accumulate in the arteries, causing clogging. When LDLs are found in the bloodstream, they usually contain about 60 to 70 percent cholesterol.

A high level of high-density lipoproteins, however, which contain only 20 to 30 percent cholesterol, is usually associated with a low-risk of developing heart disease. The role of HDL is not clear, but it is believed to transport cholesterol to the liver for resynthesis, thus helping to prevent clogging of the arteries. Compared to men, younger women usually have higher levels of HDL.

Managing your blood cholesterol level is recognized as a critical element in the fight against coronary heart disease. In some cases, drugs may be needed to lower blood cholesterol significantly, when diet alone cannot do the job. It has been demonstrated that a one-percent reduction in cholesterol level may result in a two-percent reduction in risk of heart attack.

The body's ability to manufacture cholesterol has caused some health professionals to question or minimize the role of dietary cholesterol. Many experts believe lowering saturated fat in the diet is of greater importance. Also, the effects of cigarette smoking and high blood pressure are commonly recognized for their contributions to heart attack risk.

New research is looking into whether high cholesterol levels in elderly women should be treated with low-fat diets or drugs, especially in women who are frail, undernourished, or lack variety in their diets.

The National Cholesterol Education Program (NCEP) reports that one out of four adults has a cholesterol level high enough to warrant further evaluation and, possibly, medical attention. The following chart gives the NCEP classifications of blood cholesterol levels.

National Education Cholesterol Program Classifications for Cholesterol and LDL Levels

Total Cholesterol

Under 200	desirable
200-239	borderline high
240 or more	high

LDL-Cholesterol

Under 130	desirable
130-159	borderline high
160 or more	high

What risk factors should you be concerned about?

Prior heart attack or stroke—
the most powerful risk factor.

Family history—
especially a close male family member who developed heart disease prior to age 55 or a close female relative who developed heart disease before age 65.

Women over age 54 or women with premature menopause not taking hormone replacement therapy—
Research shows that estrogen replacement therapy can reduce the risk by 44 percent. The presence of estrogen offers significant benefits to women, as evidenced by the fact that women usually develop heart disease an average of 6 to 10 years later than men. After menopause, cholesterol levels in women rise and HDL levels drop. Estrogen therapy in postmenopausal women seems to increase the HDL and decrease total cholesterol, thus protecting against heart disease.

Oral contraceptive pills—
Birth control pills were, for many years, thought to increase heart attack risk because research done in the 1960s and 1970s of women on high-dose estrogen pills seemed to have an increase in blood clots. Today, however, birth control pills provide low-dose estrogen and afford little or no risk at all.

Cigarette smoking—
Cigarette smoke has direct toxic effects on artery walls. Research shows that risk of coronary heart disease is reduced 50 to 70 percent by simply stopping smoking.

High blood pressure—
A blood pressure higher than 130 over 85 places stress on blood vessel walls increasing the risk of heart attack.

With a mere 100 calories, a medium potato contains virtually no fat, 5 grams of fiber, vitamin C, iron, niacin, and potassium.

Diabetes—

High blood sugar damages artery walls and makes platelets "stickier" and more likely to form clots. Uncontrolled diabetes often causes elevated blood fats (cholesterol and triglycerides).

Overweight—

Being more than 30 percent over ideal body weight promotes high blood pressure, diabetes, and high cholesterol. People at ideal body weight have a 35 to 55 percent lower risk for coronary heart disease.

Inactivity—

People who maintain an active lifestyle enjoy a 45 percent lower risk of heart disease than inactive people. Regular aerobic exercise helps tone the heart muscle, improves its ability to pump blood, and helps increase HDL (the good cholesterol). Exercise also helps lower blood pressure, decreases your risk for developing diabetes, and keeps your weight under control—all of which if left unchecked contribute to an increased risk for heart disease.

Diet: The Safest and Cheapest Way to Treat High Cholesterol

Many people are able to lower their cholesterol by as much as 25 percent by following a heart healthy eating plan. Here's how.

1. Reduce your total dietary fat to less than 30 percent of total daily calories.

Daily Calories	30% of Calories	Grams of Fat
1200	360	40
1500	450	50
1800	540	60
2000	600	67
2500	750	83
2700	810	90

Remember, one gram of fat has about 9 calories. To put this in perspective, one tablespoon of butter, approximately 10 grams, has about 100 calories. Based on a 2000-calories-per-day allotment, only three pats of butter a day make up about half the fat grams allowed daily. Also bear in mind that there is hidden fat in many cooked foods (although we recommend using Pam or other vegetable sprays in your pans instead of oil or butter), and, as a woman, you'll want to drink milk, eat yogurt, or have some cheese to take care of your calcium needs. All of these add to your daily fat grams total.

2. Reduce your saturated fat intake to less than 10 percent of your total daily calories.

Daily Calories	10% of Calories	Grams of Saturated Fat
1200	120	13
1500	150	16
1800	180	20
2000	200	22
2500	250	28
2700	270	30

Remember, saturated fat is part of the total fat picture. This is important when you read food labels and choose your dairy products.

3. Reduce your cholesterol to 300 milligrams per day.

4. Eat no more than 3 to 4 egg yolks per week; egg whites are okay and work well in recipes as a substitution for multiple eggs.

5. Eat less than 6 ounces cooked lean meat, fish, or poultry per day (3 ounces cooked equals the size of a deck of cards).

6. Avoid cholesterol-rich organ meats like liver, kidney, and brains.

7. Increase your intake of complex carbohydrates (whole grains, cereals, pasta, legumes).

8. Read food labels carefully.

If you are unable to lower your cholesterol in three months, the National Cholesterol Education Program recommends consulting with a registered dietitian to begin more intensive diet therapy, lowering your fat intake even more.

In the past, it was common for many women to take care of their husbands' hearts. As we enter the last half of the 1990s, we need to learn to protect our own hearts—and our family members'—with nutrition, exercise, medical care, healthy habits, and coping strategies that reduce stress and role overload.

Popular Theories about Heart Disease

The Fish-Oil Theory

Several studies in the 1980s, based on the diets of Eskimos and their low incidence of heart disease, suggested that a diet high in fish oils (known as Omega 3 fatty acids) may reduce the incidence of heart disease by causing less sticky platelets in the blood and relaxing the lining of artery walls. Additional studies have shown that while fish oils may reduce high blood pressure, they may also raise blood cholesterol.

For now, there is not sufficient evidence to suggest that much benefit accrues from taking fish-oil supplements. Women who hope to benefit from the effects of fish oil are encouraged to eat more fish, but forget the pills.

The Soluble-Fiber Theory

Soluble fiber, most notably found in oats, is also found in corn, beans, lentils, and peas. It has been shown to reduce moderately high cholesterol levels by about 20 percent, in combination with a low-fat, low-cholesterol diet. While insoluble fiber, like wheat bran, has no direct effect on cholesterol, eating soluble fiber helps reduce cholesterol in two ways: (1) by replacing high-fat foods in the diet and (2) by acting as a sponge and carrying LDL out of the body. Pectin, also a soluble fiber found in fruits such as tart apples, citrus fruit, cranberries, and sour plums, and psyllium, found in commercial bulk laxatives like Metamucil, also have a cholesterol-lowering effect. Getting your fiber from your foods is the first step before supplementation.

The Alcohol Effect Theory

People who drink moderate amounts of alcohol (one or two drinks per day) seem to have a lower rate of heart disease than non-drinkers and heavy drinkers. The exact mechanism by which this benefit results is still unknown, but if you are a moderate drinker, be aware that alcohol does contain calories, about 7 per gram. It is processed in the body just like a fat calorie.

Also, more studies are underway to solve what has become known as "The French Paradox." French men eat a very high-fat diet, but they also drink red wine with their meals. They have half the death rate from heart disease as American men. More research is needed before any conclusions can be drawn or comparisons among populations of women can be made.

Menopause

Women's bodies are constantly changing throughout their lives. At age 10, girls are considered to be pretty much alike biologically, but once puberty begins, hormonal differences begin to emerge. Through the reproductive years, these individual differences make each woman even more unique from her sisters, and by the time we reach the pre-menopausal and post-menopausal years, hardly any two of us is alike.

Women are born with all the eggs their bodies will ever produce. As we reach puberty, these eggs ripen and we begin our monthly cycles. When we begin to run out of eggs, our hormonal levels change in response to this. These are the perimenopausal years. As the supply of eggs further dwindles and our periods stop, we reach menopause. While we never really run completely out of estrogen and progesterone in our bodies, the levels wane with the diminishing egg supply and other biological systems respond.

When your periods stop, you have reached menopause. The years following menopause are known as the post-menopausal period. Those years last from one year beyond your last period until the end of your life.

Each year from here on out, based on current population levels, over one million women will reach menopause. Some 600,000 additional women will experience surgical menopause as the result of hysterectomy. Menopause itself is a perfectly natural event in the lives of women and should not be construed in any way as an illness. But it does require some special nutritional support.

Some of the common complaints some women express during the peri-menopausal years are hot flashes, sleeplessness, weight gain, and mood swings. While none of these is life-threatening, each can be somewhat inconvenient. Hormone replacement therapy helps many women, but some manage to make it comfortably through these midlife years using only nutrition and exercise.

Food to Feel Better

There is evidence that in addition to eating right, a multiple vitamin (not a megadose) taken as a supplement offers additional support during the premenopausal period. The supplement should include vitamin E and vitamin C, among others, both of which have been shown effective in alleviating hot flashes.

Some of the dietary changes you may want to incorporate into your personal healthy foodstyle are the elimination or limitation on your use of alcohol, tobacco, and caffeine, all of which can aggravate premenopausal symptoms. Use of hot drinks and spicy foods and eating large meals have been reported to trigger hot flashes for some women.

Drinking lots of water, eating smaller meals, and getting more exercise are all helpful in controlling menopause symptoms.

For years we were told that being a little plump in midlife and during menopause was beneficial. That idea is being questioned, however, in light of a recent study. As we've discussed, in a 14-year study of 116,000 women, researchers found that women who gained even 11 to 18 pounds after age 18 had a 25 percent greater chance of suffering or dying of a heart attack than women who gained less than 11 pounds. Similar gains in men may be worse, other studies show. It should be noted, however, that other variables besides weight gain, such as fitness level and family history, may have affected the results of the 116,000-women study. Severe obesity complicates menopause and causes damage to other body systems leading often to premature death, so extreme overweight should be treated medically.

Here are some foodstyle guidelines for the perimenopausal years:

- Drink lots of water: A minimum of eight 8-ounce glasses a day.
- Use sesame oil, olive, or canola oil instead of any margarine or oil containing saturated fat.
- Eat more chicken, fish, beans, legumes, and soy protein (such as tofu), and less beef and pork.
- Get enough calcium, but don't overdo dairy products. One portion is equal to 1 cup nonfat milk, 1 cup nonfat yogurt, or half a cup of nonfat or low-fat cottage cheese.
- Follow the Food Guide Pyramid Five-A-Day plan and have at least 5 servings every day of fresh fruits and vegetables.
- Eat 3 or more servings of complex carbohydrates: whole grains, dried beans, peas, and lentils, in particular.
- Be aware of your sodium intake, and try to have less than 2,400 to 3,000 milligrams a day.

Even with a healthy foodstyle, it is a good idea to consider a multiple vitamin for additional nutritional support. Supplemental calcium is also highly recommended, which you'll read more about in the discussion of osteoporosis. When selecting your multiple vitamin, be sure it is well rounded with vitamins A, B complex, C, E, and the mineral selenium.

The Value of Exercise

There is evidence that during midlife, we tend to slow down our physical activity. We are beyond the years of chasing toddlers around and spending hours at the park pushing little ones in swings. Because of this slow down, we need to eat less just to stay even in terms of our body weight. Even 100 extra calories a day can add 10 extra pounds in one year.

Regular exercise helps burn excess calories, increases your metabolic rate, and increases your overall sense of well-being. Women who follow a regular exercise program report fewer symptoms associated with menopause than women who do not exercise.

As you'll read in the section on osteoporosis, you need to work some weight-bearing exercise into your activity routine. Weight-bearing exercise includes aerobics, dancing, and walking. In short, any activity in which you bear your weight counts at this time. You need to do this to stress your skeletal structure, which in turn prompts your body to build new bone. More about this later.

Hormone Replacement Therapy

Hormone levels at menopause change dramatically for some women; particularly levels of estrogen and progesterone. While the role of these chemicals is pretty clear in terms of the menstrual cycle, their other functions remain a bit obscure.

Many women, however, are known to benefit from hormone replacement therapy. And the benefit goes beyond warding off hot flashes. As a matter of fact, today we know that estrogen is important in the prevention of osteoporosis and heart disease. If you are approaching midlife, learn all you can about menopause and discuss hormone replacement therapy with your doctor.

Osteoporosis

Osteoporosis is a bone weakening disease resulting in brittle, weak bones that are very susceptible to fracture even with normal use. Today, osteoporosis has reached epidemic proportions worldwide, and the economic costs are staggering.

All adults lose bone density as they grow older, usually beginning when they are in their 30s. But osteoporosis is of particular concern to post-menopausal, white women and older adults of both sexes. In the United States, 20 to 25 million people over the age of 45 may be afflicted. It is estimated that by age 65, one-third of all post-menopausal women and older adults will experience initial vertebral fractures. Many women do not realize they have this disease. They can lose up to 60 percent of their bone calcium by age 60 and not know it.

Osteoporosis develops slowly and often occurs in women within 10 to 15 years after their final menstrual period. This type of osteoporosis is linked to the decreased production of estrogen that coincides with menopause. It primarily affects the wrists and spine. Women are six times more likely than men to be affected by this form of osteoporosis. Sometimes the osteoporosis is accelerated due to steroid use or thyroid disease.

Senile osteoporosis results from the gradual loss of wrist, spine, and hip bone, due to decreased bone cell activity that normally accompanies aging. Inadequate calcium intake and decreased physical activity contribute to the process, which affects both men and women equally once they reach age 70.

Chronic renal disease, overactive thyroid, some forms of cancer, and some surgical procedures (like removal of the ovaries at an early age or removal of part of the stomach) can lead to bone loss, too. Some medications can also have deleterious effects on bone.

Are you at risk?

Bone mass density varies greatly from one individual to another. Genetic factors, nutritional status, lifestyle, and mechanical stress all affect bone mass density.

Osteoporosis can be detected with a quick, painless test.

For more information on bone density testing facilities, call the National Osteoporosis Foundation at (800) 464-6700.

Overall Risk Factors for Osteoporosis

- Female
- Thin, small-framed body
- Early menopause, decreased sex hormones
- Caucasian or Asian descent
- Low calcium intake
- Inactive lifestyle
- Underweight
- Family history of osteoporosis
- Heavy alcohol consumption
- Heavy cigarette smoking
- High caffeine consumption

Genetic Factors and Family History

Race—

Skeletal differences occur between races. The prevalence of osteoporosis and related fractures is higher in Caucasian and Asian women than in women of African origin. The incidence of hip fractures is approximately twice as high in white women as in black women. Osteoporosis most often affects families in which ancestors have been afflicted.

Gender—

Women have less bone mass than men at any adult age, sometimes as much as 30 percent less actual bone mass and 15 percent lower bone mass density, making them more at risk overall.

Overall, osteoporosis occurs more frequently in women than in men. Reasons for this include:

- Women tend to consume less calcium than men in their daily diets.

- Women have less bone mass due to having a smaller body size.

- Bone density loss begins earlier in women and is accelerated by changes experienced during menopause.

- Because women typically experience longer lives than men, they are more apt to encounter osteoporosis in their later years. Between the ages of 45 and 75, women lose almost one-third of their bone mass, mostly because of the reduced production of the hormone estrogen.

Nutritional Status

Calcium—

Adequate calcium intake is especially important in the bone-building years of childhood, adolescence, and the senior adult years. During childhood and adolescence, a large amount of calcium is absorbed by the bones. The Recommended Dietary Allowance for calcium (1200 milligrams—equivalent to about 3 to 4 servings of dairy products per day) was recently extended to age 24, particularly to encourage peak bone mass building in young women.

Elderly adults, on the other hand, need to consume adequate calcium in order to slow down age-related bone loss. Recommendations range from 1000 milligrams of calcium per day for pre-menopausal women to 1500 milligrams a day for elderly women not taking estrogen.

Many other nutrients besides calcium affect the absorption of calcium and the development of bone mass. Vitamins A, C, D, and many minerals affect bone metabolism and calcium balance. During the winter, women living in cold, less-sunny climates usually receive insufficient amounts of vitamin D, the sunshine vitamin. Diets that include too much protein or sodium (salt) and too little calcium can cause calcium to be excreted by the body instead of used. Other lifestyle factors also play a role in keeping bones strong and healthy.

Lifestyle Factors

Alcohol—
High alcohol consumption is thought to limit bone formation. Alcoholics have an increased risk of fracture and reduced bone density. Much of the reason for this could stem from the fact that diets of heavy drinkers are often lacking in calcium, minerals, vitamin D, and protein.

Smoking—
Heavy smokers have significantly lower bone mass density than non-smokers; many maintain a lean body weight and experience an accelerated rate of post-menopausal bone loss. Women smokers have experienced an increase in hip fractures as a result.

Caffeine—
Because caffeine increases the excretion of calcium by the body, use of caffeinated products should be limited. That means cutting back on coffee, tea, and caffeinated soft drinks.

Mechanical Stress

Inactivity and prolonged bed rest directly result in bone loss. This explains why athletes have a higher bone mass than non-athletes. Obese women have one-third the risk of developing osteoporosis than extremely thin women, probably because extra weight helps preserve bone mass.

Health and Medical Factors

Amenorrhea (lack of menstrual periods) is associated with low bone mass density. Women athletes (with amenorrhea) who engage in endurance activity may have as much as 22 to 30 percent less bone mass density than other women their age.

Treating Osteoporosis

Making some simple changes in your foodstyle and lifestyle can help prevent future fractures, even if you have already developed a fracture as the result of osteoporosis. A diet rich in calcium, frequent weight-bearing exercise (approved by your doctor), training in fall prevention, and use of hormone replacement therapy or new drug treatments may all help to minimize the consequences of osteoporosis or bring it under control.

Calcium is needed for strong bones. It is also an important mineral for the heart, muscles, nerves, and blood clotting. All of the calcium in the world by itself will not protect anyone against bone loss caused by estrogen deficiency, inactivity, excessive smoking, alcohol use, or various medical disorders and their treatments, however. Calcium is just one of the pieces needed for a healthy skeleton and healthy bone mass.

Lack of calcium is thought to play a major role in the development of osteoporosis. Unlike some other nutrients, the human body does not make calcium on its own. Many women and adolescent girls consume only half the recommended calcium needed for the growth and maintenance of healthy bones. It is during certain times in a woman's life—childhood, adolescence, pregnancy, and during lactation—that the body's demand for calcium is greatest.

The recommended daily calcium intake is as follows:

Infants	*Mg Calcium per day*
birth to 6 months	400
6 months to 1 year	600
Children and young adults	
1 to 10 years	800
11 to 24 years	1200
Adults	
25 and over	800
Females over 50 years who take estrogen	1000
Females over 50 years who do not take estrogen	1500
Pregnant and lactating women	1200

Although many women think of milk and dairy products when they think of calcium, there are many other food sources that contribute calcium to the diet. Refer to the following chart for calcium-rich food sources.

Good Food Sources of Calcium

Food Item	Serving Size	Calcium (mg)
Milk		
whole	1 cup	291
2%	1 cup	295
skim	1 cup	302
Yogurt (with added milk solids)		
plain, low fat	1 cup	415
fruited, low fat	1 cup	343
frozen, fruit-flavored	1 cup	240
frozen, chocolate	1 cup	160
Custard, baked	1/2 cup	150
Pudding	1/2 cup	135
Cheese		
mozzarella, part skim	1 ounce	207
Swiss	1 ounce	207
muenster	1 ounce	203
cheddar	1 ounce	204
ricotta, part skim	1/2 cup	335
cottage, low fat	1/2 cup	78
macaroni and cheese	1/2 cup	180

Good Food Sources of Calcium, continued

Food Item	Serving Size	Calcium (mg)
Ice cream, vanilla		
hard	1/2 cup	90
soft	1/2 cup	120
Ice milk, vanilla		
hard	1/2 cup	88
soft	1/2 cup	137
Seafood		
oysters, raw (13-19)	1 cup	226
sardines, in oil, drained, with bones	3 ounces	372
salmon, pink, canned, with bones	3 ounces	167
shrimp, canned, drained	3 ounces	96
Vegetables		
kale, raw	1 cup	180
bok choy, raw	1 cup	74
broccoli, fresh cooked	1 cup	136
broccoli, frozen cooked	1 cup	100
collard greens, fresh cooked	1 cup	357
turnip greens, fresh cooked	1 cup	252
soybeans, cooked	1 cup	131

Good Food Sources of Calcium, continued

Food Item	Serving Size	Calcium (mg)
Tofu	1/2 cup	50 to 250
Almonds	1 ounce	75
Bread, fortified with calcium	1 slice	290
Cereal, fortified with calcium	1 ounce	310
Juice/drink, fortified with calcium	1 cup	300

Lactose Intolerance

Some people can't digest milk properly and suffer stomach upset, diarrhea, gas, and bloating. This is referred to as lactose intolerance. Those who suffer this intolerance lack the enzyme "lactase" that is needed to break down milk sugar. For them, milk is difficult to tolerate; however, some people who are lactose intolerant can eat yogurt and hard cheese without problems. There are alternative milks, too, such as acidophilus milk and commercial milk, products in which the milk sugar has been treated. Tablets and drops are available that can be added to milk to break down the lactose in the milk, neutralizing the lactose. All the foods listed in the chart as sources of calcum are good alternatives to milk for those who cannot comfortably consume it.

Factors that Affect Calcium Absorption

Certain components of food can affect how much calcium is absorbed or excreted by the body. More research is needed, but excessive amounts of caffeine, protein, and salt are known to retard calcium absorption. Vitamin D and milk sugar (lactose), on the other hand, enhance calcium absorption.

Calcium Supplements

If you think you need to supplement your calcium intake, contact your doctor or a pharmacist before making your supplement selection. Of course, the amount of supplemental calcium you need will depend in large part on how much dietary calcium you are getting in your food, plus the other factors mentioned above: your age and hormonal status.

There are a variety of supplements available, but they are not all of equal value. The most common supplements are calcium carbonate, calcium citrate, calcium lactate, and calcium gluconate. Studies done during the late 1980s showed that calcium citrate was absorbed better than the other forms of calcium, particularly in people with low levels of stomach acid, a condition common in women over age 40.

Reading labels is important because the amount of elemental calcium, that is the amount of calcium that is actually available to your body, depends on the form of the calcium compound that is used. Here's how they rate:

Calcium carbonate—40 percent

Calcium citrate—24 percent

Calcium lactate—13 percent

Calcium gluconate—9 percent

Here's how it works: If the label on your calcium carbonate supplement says 1,000 milligrams, you will actually get only 40 percent of elemental calcium, or 400 milligrams. The other 600 milligrams is the carbonate part.

Remember, food is your best source of calcium, but when you fall short in your diet or if your calories don't allow, take a supplement.

Tips on Taking Calcium Supplements

When taking a calcium supplement, you need to know that absorption is enhanced when you take it with a small amount of milk or yogurt. These foods contain vitamin D and milk sugar, both of which improve your body's reception to the supplemental calcium.

If you wonder whether you are absorbing the calcium tablet you are taking, here's a quick test: Place the tablet in 6 ounces of vinegar at room temperature. Stir occasionally and observe for 30 minutes. If the tablet has not dissolved after 30 minutes, it is not easily digestible in your system. Discard it and try another brand.

If you take calcium carbonate, take it at mealtime. Other forms should be taken at bedtime and usually with milk or yogurt. They also act as a mild sedative and encourage sleep.

Avoid taking calcium at the same time as you take an iron supplement. The two inhibit the effectiveness of each other.

Avoid taking large doses of supplemental calcium all at once. Take 500 milligrams or less at a time because it is best absorbed if taken in smaller amounts throughout the day. Taking more than 2500 milligrams per day may cause the formation of kidney stones, so be cautious.

Avoid calcium pills made from dolomite or bone meal because they may contain lead or other toxic metals.

Avoid taking calcium with high-fiber meals or bulk-forming laxatives (like Metamucil) because fiber may reduce calcium absorption.

Drink plenty of fluids when you take supplements of any kind.

Look for calcium-fortified foods (juices, cereals, breads) as an alternative to calcium tablets.

Exercise

Exercise makes bones stronger. Exercise may increase peak bone mass in younger women and decrease bone loss in older women. Weight bearing exercises, such as walking, jogging, stair climbing, and hiking, are recommended over swimming or biking because the mechanical stress they exert on bones promotes bone formation.

Hormone Replacement Therapy in Osteoporosis

Supplemental estrogen is often recommended for post-menopausal women since estrogen is known to have some calcium-retaining effect on bones among this population. Osteoporosis can be prevented or postponed in some women who opt for hormone replacement therapy. Discuss all the options with your physician if you are at risk.

Premenstrual Syndrome (PMS)

In the last ten years, we have begun to come to grips with the hormonal shifts that precipitate PMS. It is estimated that 40 percent of all women between the ages of 14 and 50 experience the symptoms that describe premenstrual syndrome. At least 10 percent of these women experience symptoms severe enough to disrupt their daily activities.

Symptoms of PMS affect emotional, physical, and psychological aspects of women's lives. While the specific symptoms vary from woman to woman, all women share one common element: the time during the cycle when these symptoms occur. This is usually 2 to 14 days prior to a woman's menstrual period. Symptoms subsequently disappear after the period begins. Women with true PMS usually also experience a symptom-free time sometime during the monthly cycle. As many as 150 symptoms have been identified in PMS. Here are the most common: weight gain, irritability, anxiety, depression, fluid retention, backache, abdominal bloating, breast tenderness and swelling, craving for sweets or alcohol or salt, other appetite changes, fatigue, constipation, and acne.

Why do we suffer PMS?

The causes of PMS have yet to be identified, but are probably related to the hormonal shifts that occur during the menstrual cycle. Some causes that have been theorized include:

- vitamin or mineral deficiencies (particularly low levels of vitamin B)
- poor diet or other nutritional factors
- hypoglycemia (low blood sugar)
- progesterone deficiency (progesterone is an important female hormone)
- fluid retention
- excessive levels of prolactin (a pituitary hormone)
- stress

Without full understanding of the cause, medical treatments are not yet totally defined. However, diet, exercise, vitamin and mineral supplements, stress reduction, and sedative-style medications may all be recommended by your physician.

Diagnosis of PMS is best made by the woman who experiences it. There are as yet no laboratory tests to confirm it. Keeping a daily record of when your symptoms occur for at least three full cycles can help you and your doctor determine what should be done.

How can diet help?

Eating a well balanced diet can supply adequate vitamins and minerals. Special vitamin and mineral supplements are available. Excessive amounts of vitamin B6 should be avoided since toxic effects have been shown to cause irreversible nerve damage.

Eating six small meals a day instead of three large ones can help maintain steady energy levels and avoid energy highs and lows.

Eating more complex carbohydrates (vegetables, fruits, whole grains, and legumes: dried beans and peas) and cutting back on simple carbohydrates (refined sugar, soft drinks, and sweets) helps.

Limit your caffeine to help reduce feelings of nervousness.

Limit your alcohol intake to stave off depression.

Limit your salt intake to avoid fluid retention.

Can exercise help with PMS?

Regular exercise (at least 3 times per week for 20 to 30 minutes) can help alleviate the symptoms of PMS. It improves blood circulation, reduces stress and muscle tension, and provides you with an overall sense of well being.

While there is no single therapy that works for all women, managing your diet, getting regular exercise, and talking with your physician about a medication that might be right for you are all good approaches to managing PMS.

Foods to Stay Vibrant, Young & Healthy

Appendix

Water-Soluble Vitamins

Vitamin—C, Ascorbic Acid

What it does—Promotes healthy gums and teeth, aids in iron absorption, and aids body in forming collagen, the basis of connective tissue. Antioxidant.

Where to get it—Fresh fruits (particularly citrus fruits) and vegetables: oranges, sprouts, strawberries, broccoli, tomatoes, sweet potatoes, cantaloupe

How much do you need?—60 mg/day

Vitamin—B1, Thiamin

What it does—Needed for breakdown of carbohydrates for energy. Necessary for healthy brain and nerve cells and heart functioning.

Where to get it—Pork, lean meats, fish, oranges, dried beans and peas, wheat germ, whole grains, pasta

How much do you need?—1.1 mg/day

Vitamin—B2, Riboflavin

What it does—Essential for normal release of energy. Aids normal growth, production, and regulation of certain hormones, and formation of red blood cells.

Where to get it—Milk, milk products, lean meats, eggs, green leafy vegetables, legumes, enriched breads and cereals

How much do you need?—1.3 mg/day

Vitamin—B3, Niacin

What it does—Important in release of energy from carbohydrates. Maintains functioning of skin, nerve, and digestive system.

Where to get it—Dairy products, lean meats, chicken, fish, cooked dried beans and peas, soybeans, nuts, peanuts, legumes, enriched breads and cereals

How much do you need?—15 mg/day

Vitamin—B5, Pantothenic Acid

What it does—Acts as catalyst in conversion of fats, carbohydrates, and protein to energy. Essential for metabolizing food and in the synthesis of various body chemicals, such as hormones and cholesterol

Where to get it—Liver, fish, chicken, eggs, whole grain breads, cereals, dried beans, nuts, dates, potatoes

How much do you need?—No recommended daily dietary allowance has been established, although 4 to 7 mg/day has been estimated as safe and adequate.

Vitamin—B6, Pyridoxine

What it does—Important in chemical reactions of protein and protein components. Helps maintain normal brain functioning and aids in formation of red blood cells.

Where to get it—Lean meat, wheat germ, brewer's yeast, poultry, fish, soybeans, cooked dried beans and peas, peanuts

How much do you need?—1.6 mg/day

Vitamin—Biotin

What it does—Helps metabolize amino acids and carbohydrates.

Where to get it—Liver, eggs, soybeans, peanuts, yeast, milk, milk products

How much do you need?—No recommended daily dietary allowance has been established, although 30 to 100 mcg/day has been estimated as safe and adequate.

Vitamin—Folacin (folic acid)

What it does—Important in synthesis of DNA, necessary for new cell and protein synthesis, and works with vitamin B12. Vital to normal growth and cell maintenance.

Where to get it—Wheat bran, beans, dark leafy vegetable, liver

How much do you need?—180 mcg/day

Vitamin—B12, Cobalamin

What it does—Aids in formation and maintenance of central nervous system. Helps manufacture red blood cells.

Where to get it—Lean meat, poultry, fish, shellfish, liver, eggs, milk, milk products

How much do you need?—2 mcg/day

Fat-Soluble Vitamins

Vitamin—A

What it does—Promotes good vision and maintains healthy skin, teeth, skeletal tissue. Beta carotene converts to vitamin A in body. Antioxidant.

Where to get it—Liver, eggs, fortified milk, dark green, yellow, and orange vegetables, spinach, carrots, sweet potatoes, apricots, peaches, cantaloupe

How much do you need?—800 mcg retinol equivalents*/day

Vitamin—D

What it does—Can be produced in the body from exposure to sunlight. Promotes calcium absorption for healthy bones and teeth.

Where to get it—Fortified milk, butter, margarine, cheese, fish, fortified cereals, sunlight

How much do you need?—5 mcg or 200 IU/day

1 retinol equivalent equals 1 mcg retinol or 6 mcg beta carotene

Vitamin—E

What it does—Antioxidant. Protects tissue from oxidation via free radicals. Important in formation of red blood cells; helps body use vitamin K.

Where to get it—Vegetable oils, wheat germ, nuts, whole grains, asparagus, spinach

How much do you need?—8 mg/day

Vitamin—K

What it does—Regulates blood clotting by aiding in production of prothrombin.

Where to get it—Green leafy vegetables: broccoli, turnip greens, romaine lettuce, cabbage; cereals, soybeans, vegetable oils

How much do you need?—65 mcg/day

Minerals—Major Minerals

Mineral—Sodium, Potassium, Chloride

What it does—

Sodium helps regulate water balance and blood pressure.

Potassium helps regulate water balance and blood pressure. Promotes regular heartbeat and is essential for muscle contraction.

Chloride helps maintain body's fluid and balances blood acid-base balance.

Where to get it—

Sodium: table salt, baking soda

Potasssium: lean meat, potatoes, avocados, bananas, apricots, orange juice, dried or fresh fruit

Chloride: table salt, fish

How much do you need?—

Sodium: 2400 to 3000 mcg/day

Potassium: No recommended dietary allowance established

Chloride: No recommended dietary allowance established

Mineral—Calcium

What it does—Works to develop and maintain health of bones and teeth. Needed for blood clotting. Helps regulate heart beat, muscle contraction, and nerve conduction.

Where to get it—Milk and milk products, canned sardines, salmon, dark green leafy vegetables

How much do you need?—800 to 1500 mg/day

Mineral—Phosphorus

What it does—Aids in bone growth. Important in energy production.

Where to get it—Meat, fish, poultry, eggs, milk and milk products, peas, beans, nuts

How much do you need?—800 mg/day

Mineral—Magnesium

What it does—Aids in bone growth and in function of nerves and muscles.

Where to get it—Nuts, cooked dried beans and peas, soy beans, whole grain breads and cereals, wheat bran, dark green leafy vegetables, seafood, bananas, apricots

How much do you need?—280 mg/day

Minerals—Trace Minerals

Mineral—Iron

What it does—Essential to formation of hemoglobin, which carries oxygen in the blood, and myoglobin which carries oxygen in muscles.

Where to get it—Organ meats, lean red meat, egg yolks, dried fruits, cooked dried beans and peas, green leafy vegetables, prune juice, oysters, enriched grain products

How much do you need?—10 to 15 mg/day

Mineral—Zinc

What it does—Maintains taste and smell acuity. Important for cell growth and proper functioning of the immune system.

Where to get it—Oysters, lean meat, poultry, fish, whole grain breads and cereals

How much do you need?—12 mg/day

Mineral—Iodine

What it does—Necessary for normal function of the thyroid gland. Important for normal cell function.

Where to get it—Iodized salt, fresh-water shellfish, seafood

How much do you need?—150 mcg/day

Mineral—Copper

What it does—Helps in the formation of red blood cells. Keeps bones, blood vessels, nerves, and immune system healthy.

Where to get it—Whole grain breads and cereals, shellfish, nuts, organ meats, poultry, cooked dried beans and peas, dark green leafy vegetable

How much do you need?—No recommended daily dietary allowance has been established, although 1.5 to 3 mg/day has been estimated as safe and adequate.

Mineral—Manganese

What it does—Necessary for normal bone growth and development and cell function and reproduction.

Where to get it—Spinach, tea, whole grain breads and cereals, raisins, blueberries, wheat bran, pineapple, nuts, cocoa powder

How much do you need?—No recommended daily dietary allowance has been established, although 2 to 5 mg/day has been estimated as safe and adequate.

Mineral—Fluoride

What it does—Important for dental and bone health.

Where to get it—Fluoridated water, fish, tea, gelatin

How much do you need?—No recommended daily dietary allowance has been established, although 1.5 to 4 mg/day has been estimated as safe and adequate.

Mineral—Chromium

What it does—Component of glucose tolerance factor that works with insulin for uptake of blood sugar for energy.

Where to get it—Whole grain breads and cereals, pork kidneys, molasses, lean meats, cheese, dried beans and peas, peanuts

How much do you need?—No recommended daily dietary allowance has been established, although 50 to 200 mg/day has been estimated as safe and adequate.

Mineral—Selenium

What it does—Component of powerful antioxidant enzyme that protects red blood cells and cell membranes.

Where to get it—Grains grown in selenium-rich soil, seafood, poultry, red meat, egg yolks, tuna, garlic, tomatoes

How much do you need?—55 mcg/day

Mineral—Molybdenum

What it does—Vital to normal cell function for normal growth and development.

Where to get it—Lean meat, whole grain breads and cereals, cooked dried beans and peas, dark green leafy vegetables, organ meats

How much do you need?—No recommended daily dietary allowance has been established, although 75 to 250 mg/day has been estimated as safe and adequate.

Index

effects of added weight, 59
reducing risk of, 7, 8
sunlight and skin, 190
canned foods, purchasing, 152
canola oil, 9
cantaloupe, 1, 147
carbohydrates, 6-7, 9, 22, 23, 35
calorie content of, 64
fast-acting, 196
types of, 7-8
cardiovascular disease, 202-210
and exercise, 81
reducing risks of, 8
carrots, 1, 7
casseroles, reducing fat in, 86
cellulose, 35
cereal, purchasing, 145
CFS (chronic fatigue syndrome), 195
cheddar cheese, purchasing, 142
Chinese food, 162-163, 166
chips, preparing, 145
chloride, 10, 45, 233-234
cholesterol, 31-34
and heart disease, 134, 203-204
blood, reducing, 7
content of foods, 32-34
effects of fiber, 36
free, defined, 132
guidelines, 208
intake, recommended amount, 31
recommended levels of, 204
reducing, 1, 205
choosing healthy foods, 3
chromium, 10, 237
chronic fatigue syndrome, 195
clothing, exercise, 90
cobalamin, 10, 232
cobalt, 10

cocktails, calorie content of, 161
coffee, 53-55
cola drinks, 53-55
cold cuts, fat content, 144
colitis, 36
colon cancer, 12
fiber and, 36
complete protein, defined, 8
complex carbohydrates, 7-8, 12, 35
complications, diabetes, 198-199
condiments, 165
conditioning, 82
constipation, 10
and fiber, 36, 201
contains, defined, 131
cookies, purchasing, 153
cooking spray, 53
cooking techniques, 11, 82
copper, 10, 236
Council of Better Business Bureaus, 177
crackers, 145
cramps, muscle, 13
creamed, defined, 159
crispbread, 145
crispy, defined, 159
croissants, 145, 166
cross country ski machines, 97
cruciferous vegetables, 191
cruise meals, 169
cyclamates, 43

daily values, food label, 126-127
dairy products, purchasing, 142-143
dancing, 83
decaffeinated beverages, 56
deli products, purchasing, 143
dental caries, effects of sugar, 41

hypertension
  and exercise, 81
  and sodium, 135
  effects of added weight, 59
  effects of salt, 45
hypoglycemia, 196, 198
hysterectomy, 211

ice cream, purchasing, 146
iceberg lettuce, 70
impaired glucose tolerance, 198
incomplete protein, defined, 8
insulin, 195
  resistance, 197
insulin-dependent diabetes mellitus, 195-197
insuluble fiber, 35-36
intensity, exercise, 92-94
iodine, 10, 236
iron, 10, 12, 24, 235
  deficiency, 184-187
  recommended levels, 185
iron-rich foods, 185
isoleucine, 9
Italian food, 163

jogging, 83
juice, fruit, purchasing, 146
jumping rope, 83

kidney disease and hypertension,
  45

labels, food, 126-136
lactation and caffeine, 54
lactose, 7
  intolerance, 222
large bowel cancer, 36
LDL cholesterol, 28, 203

lean, defined, 132
legumes, 7
less, defined, 131
lettuce, 70
leucine, 9
lifestyle, changing your, 2
light salts, 49
light, defined, 131
lignin, 35
linoleic acid, 10, 30
linolenic acid, 10, 30
lipoproteins, 31, 203
lite, defined, 131
low calorie, defined, 132
low cholesterol, defined, 132
low fat, defined, 132
low saturated fat, defined, 132
low sodium, defined, 132
low-density lipoprotein cholesterol (LDL), 31, 203
low-fat foods, 30
  calorie content of, 64-65
lunch meats, fat content, 144
lysine, 9

macaroni and cheese, 8
magnesium, 10, 235
major minerals, 10, 233-235
maltitol, 7, 42, 44
maltose, 7
mammograms, 194
manganese, 10, 236
mannitol, 7, 42, 44
margarine,
  calorie content, 29
  cholesterol content of, 65
  purchasing, 142
  water content of, 90
mayonnaise, calorie content of, 29

benzoate, 45
bicarbonate, 45
content of foods, 46-49
hidden sources of, 45
intake, recommended level, 45
products, reduced, 177
soft drinks, 165
soluble fiber, 35-36
content of foods, 40
theory, 209-210
sorbitol, 7, 42, 44
soups, selecting, 161
soy products, health benefits of, 201
soy sauce, 166
soybean curd, 146
soybeans, 7
spices, 49-51
spinach, 1, 52
Sprinkle Sweet, 44
stair climbing, 83, 97
starches, 7-8, 35
stationary bicycles, 97-98
steroids and diabetes, 198
stomach ulcers and caffeine, 53
strawberries, 1, 139, 171
strength training, 84
stress test, exercise, 87
stretching, 84-85
stroke and hypertension, 45
sucrose, 7
Sugar Twin, 44
sugar, 7, 25, 35, 40-42
alcohols, 7, 42, 44
free, defined, 132
intake, recommended level, 41
other names for, 41-42
sugar-free desserts, 146
sulfides, 191

sulfur, 10
Sunette, 43
sunlight and skin cancer, 190
supplements, 11, 13
Sweet 'n Low, 44
Sweet One, 43
sweet potatoes, 1
sweeteners, 42-44
swimming, 83
syrup, 7

tea, 53-55
thiamin, 10, 11, 229
threonine, 9
tin, 10
tips, nutrition, 26
tofu, 146, 201
tomatoes, purchasing, 139
tooth decay, effects of sugar, 41
tortillas, 145
trace minerals, 10, 235-238
traveling, eating, 168-170
treadmills, 96-97
tryptophan, 9
tuna, purchasing, 80
turkey, ground, 141
type I diabetes, 195-197
type II diabetes, 197

ulcers and caffeine, 53
underweight, problems with being, 27
unit pricing, 130
US Department of Agriculture, 18, 192

vacation, eating, 170
valine, 9